The Teacher Pr

in

Health Visiting and the Social Services

Second Edition

Peter Jarvis and Sheila Gibson

Department of Educational Studies
University of Surrey

Stanley Thornes (Publishers) Ltd

First published in 1985 by Chapman & Hall
(ISBN 0–412–34010–0)

Second edition published in 1997 by:
Stanley Thornes (Publishers) Ltd
Ellenborough House
Wellington Street
CHELTENHAM
GL50 1YW
United Kingdom

97 98 99 00 01 / 10 9 8 7 6 5 4 3 2 1

A catalogue record for this book is available from the British Library.

ISBN 0–7487–3338–8

Typeset by Florencetype Ltd, Stoodleigh, Devon

Printed and bound in Great Britain by
TJ International, Padstow, Cornwall

Contents

Tables and figures

LIST OF TABLES

LIST OF FIGURES

Introduction to the second edition

The first edition of this book appeared 12 years ago and there have been so many changes since that time that the publishers asked us to revise it for a second edition. We are grateful to them for this suggestion and have gladly undertaken it, but these transformations in society have been so great that much of the book bears little resemblance to the first edition. Among the changes that we have had to take into consideration have been: the emergence of the market philosophy in both education and the health services with all its accompanying problems and rhetoric; the globalization of society and the effects of the global market on Western societies; the movement of most forms of health service education into higher education; the changing system of higher education in the United Kingdom with the introduction of a mass system of higher education; the growing significance of the postmodern debate with its accompanying changes in our understanding of society. Each of these changes impacts upon the other and society has undergone quite a profound metamorphosis in these past years. Consequently, the revision to this book has been quite radical in places.

Nevertheless, the original edition did anticipate the direction some of these changes would take. Teacher practitioners or lecturer practitioners, or mentors, etc. were not as numerous when this book appeared as they are now. It has been recognized that it is necessary to develop an understanding of practical knowledge and that the body of theory cannot stand isolated from practice, so that this bridging role is more important than ever before.

There are an increasing number of teaching/facilitating roles that seek to blur any divide between theory and practice, since one of the features of contemporary society is that boundaries are crossed and even disappear in places. This book has been written for these people: nurse and midwife teachers having a clinical role in practice, whether it be in hospital or the community; practitioners in social and community work with an educational function; those who supervize or mentor students; preceptors, etc. Indeed, there are now many who occupy these roles.

It is also written for those teachers of theory who need to understand the significance of having theories of practice and practical knowledge and who need to understand the art of teaching in an interpersonal relationship in a practical setting. Many of these teachers recognize the profound relevance of this role, something this book merely reinforces.

The main aim of the book is to provide information and ideas about teaching and learning in situations where one teacher is involved with one student, or at most with a small group of students. Individualized teaching and learning is used in this book to refer to the teaching and learning transaction where two people interact. A theoretical basis is developed here that not only relates to the teaching and learning interaction, but seeks to locate it within the changing social context, and the opening and closing chapters reflect these social transformations.

The first chapter introduces readers to the concepts of field of practice and practical knowledge and, consequently, lays a theoretical foundation for the remainder of the book. The following one seeks to highlight the essence of the teaching and learning interaction, as a relationship requiring certain skills. The next three chapters outline some of the main elements in learning and teaching in an interpersonal situation. These chapters form the core of the text. Chapter 6 examines the process of assessment, an area that causes many teacher practitioners a great deal of concern. The penultimate chapter seeks to locate this process in the wider field of higher education, while the final chapter locates it within the wider changes in society.

There is a sense in which the book is now more theoretical than the original edition and this is because professional preparation has, paradoxically, assumed a more theoretical perspective whilst endeavouring to focus more on the practical. The theory of the practical has not been developed to any great extent in vocational education, although this is emerging.

The terms teacher practitioner and mentor are used throughout this book, although it is recognized that other terms could have been employed just as usefully. It should be noted that, for consistency, the female gender is used most frequently throughout the text to refer to teachers and learners, although the male gender would have been just as appropriate in many instances.

Once again, we hope that this edition will be interesting to those who read it and, even more significantly, practical for those who use it.

The roles of the teacher practitioner and mentor

1

This chapter explores:
- *The concepts of field of practice and practical knowledge*
- *The mentor*
- *The teacher*
- *Straddling two professionalisms*
- *The teacher practitioner within professional education and training.*

INTRODUCTION

Contemporary society is one in which the practical is being increasingly emphasized, almost at the expense of the theoretical which is being reduced in some instances to 'the merely academic'. While this is not a position adopted in this book, the significance of the practical is emphasized and its relationship to the theoretical is explored in considerable detail, since this underlies the theory of the role of the teacher practitioner and the mentor. However, nursing, midwifery and health visiting have always emphasized the practical side of their work, having introduced such roles as clinical tutor, practical work teacher and field-work teacher long before many other occupations and professions had even considered the idea, although the concept of apprenticeship (*apprendre* (Fr.) = to learn) was jettisoned before it was thoroughly explored.

The title teacher practitioner is, in a sense, an umbrella term for all of these other roles which emerged in the early 1980s, encompassing the designated roles of a practitioner with a teaching responsibility in nursing, midwifery and health visiting. More recently the words have been reversed, with the appearance of practitioner teacher. Lecturer practitioner has assumed some currency since the preparation for these professions has been relocated in higher education. Nevertheless, the term teacher practitioner is used throughout this book since the meaning of the term lecturer is much more restricted than that of teacher. The use of the word lecturer in this context, however, probably reflects the higher status of a lecturer in higher education compared with that of the school teacher – although university teacher is the traditional term for one who lectures in a university. The fact that the job title changes periodically to reflect the contemporary social situation is interesting, although it can lead to some confusion.

Irrespective of the term, teacher practitioners are practitioners who have a teaching role, working in a practical setting and combining their practice with teaching the practical component of a professional role. While it might be justifiably claimed that every qualified professional has this duty, and the English National Board (ENB) requires all teachers in these professional groups to work within a practice setting for one day per week (ENB, 1993: 2.13, para 3.2), there are certain roles where the duty is particularly specified by reason of the designation and specification of the post.

In precisely the same way, another term has come to the fore in recent years, mentor, and this is also frequently used in a similar manner to teacher practitioner (see Morton-Cooper and Palmer, 1993), although its usage varies with different occupational groupings. It is similar to the teacher practitioner in as much as the mentor is usually a highly qualified professional who enters a one-to-one relationship of teaching and learning with junior colleagues in order to help them perform their role better or develop and mature as human beings.

While some of these different occupational roles are referred to in this introduction, such as clinical tutor and practical work teacher, the role of the teacher practitioner is to 'plan and provide a learning environment in the context of the specialist area of practice' (ENB, 1993: 4.35. Para 1.1).

While community mental handicap nurses (CMHNs), community psychiatric nurses (CPNs), district nurses (DNs), registered health visitors (RHVs) and occupational health nurses (OHNs) are required to study and pass a community practice teacher course comprising theory-practice components relating to teaching, learning and assessment before assuming the role of practitioner teacher, this is not the case for all teacher practitioners. Since 1992, as a result of a Joint Practice Teacher Initiative, the Community Practice Teacher Course has had to include a common core element agreed between the ENB and the Central Council for the Education and Training of Social Workers (CCETSW) and the College of Occupational Therapists (COT) (ENB, 1993: 4.35, para 1.2).

During the 1970s, according to Kadushin (1976 pp2–3) a greater emphasis was placed on the preparation of professionally trained social workers for supervision, consultation, administration and planning. According to her (Kadushin, 1976 p125):

Educational supervision is the second principal responsibility of the supervisor. Educational supervision is concerned with teaching the worker what he needs to know in order to do his job and helping him to learn . . .

This trend has continued throughout the 1980s and 1990s and it has become more formalized in the UK and USA.

Yet this teaching role has been strangely neglected by many other professions and occupations, learners being treated rather like apprentices, observing the masters at work and seeking to emulate their practice. Some branches of nursing have been much more far-sighted than this, creating both a practical teaching role and providing opportunity for some experienced practitioners to be prepared for it. The extent to which the training is adequate remains largely unresearched, although Battle and Salter (1981 p20) discovered that the practical work teachers that they interviewed were mainly satisfied with their preparation. However, there is a need for more research into the preparation of teacher practitioners in a variety of situations.

Mentors, on the other hand, have not always been trained for their role and, while some branches of nursing have used the term mentor in relation to the initial preparation of student nurses and, on occasions, for post registration students, its use is much wider in other occupations. Many professional groups have used the term to refer to a senior colleague who is given, or has assumed, some responsibility to help newly qualified employees establish themselves in the profession or the company. Occasionally, the term has also been used to describe a supervisory role.

Thus it may be seen that both teacher practitioners and mentors have a dual role: as practitioners and as teachers. But the roles may be full-time in themselves: nursing and social work are certainly full-time and so may teaching adults be a full-time occupation. Significantly the ENB requires institutions to count teachers as 0.8 full-time-equivalent in order to enable them to practise (ENB, 1993 pp2–3, para 3.2). Even so many of these teachers still have difficulty in finding time to practise their discipline on the wards or in the community, simply because of the heavy demands of their teaching role. It is also significant that school teacher trainers are also increasingly being asked to have recent and relevant school experience. Nevertheless, the roles of teacher, practitioner and mentor are very significant ones, since they are at the interface of theory and practice.

Neither the teacher practitioner's role, nor that of the mentor, are merely amalgams of the two roles that describe teacher and practitioner, they are important specialist functions in their own right. The roles of the teacher practitioner and mentor, consequently constitute the focus of this opening chapter, whilst subsequent ones develop the educational theory underlying the teaching aspect of the roles. Neither is any attempt made in this short text to discuss the occupational roles specific to the branch of nursing or social work within which the teacher practitioners and mentors may function.

THE CONCEPTS OF THE FIELD OF PRACTICE AND PRACTICAL KNOWLEDGE

A field of practice is, as the term implies, a site in which a specialist occupation is conducted. It constitutes a focus for the practice of an occupation or a profession. By contrast, a field of study is the focus of a special area of research, and in studying an occupation a field of practice for the practitioner becomes a field of study for the researcher.

Since both nursing and social work are practical professions, it seems obvious to refer to the field of nursing practice and the field of social work practice. However, professions are rarely single or simple entities, but rather they comprise a number of different strands undertaking similar work in the same or different locations. Consequently, it is more accurate to see nursing spanning a number of different fields of practice and social work doing the same. The fields within nursing and social work all overlap which suggests that there is some commonality about them, although there are are whole elements of practice which are discrete, as Figure 1.1 illustrates.

Even more significantly, some of the fields of practice of nursing may overlap with those of social work and so the occupational picture becomes even more complex. Such overlap within and between occupations reflects the fragmented world of late modern society.

Each occupation, however, has its own expertise and its own body of knowledge, so that it is easier to concentrate upon only one occupation

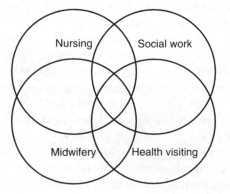

Figure 1.1 Overlapping fields of practice

in order to explore the idea of practical knowledge. Before this is undertaken, however, it is necessary to examine the idea of knowledge itself and its relation to skill. Precisely what is knowledge? How can people be sure that what they know corresponds with the 'real' world out there? How can they be sure that that knowledge is true? These are but some of the major questions that confront any philosopher analyzing knowledge itself. They cannot all be answered here since this is not the purpose of this book, but these are some of the questions that need to be explored if practical knowledge is to be understood.

Sheffler (1965) sought to respond to the questions about knowledge as truth propositions when he distinguished between three ways of verifying knowledge: rational-logical, empirical and pragmatic. Rational-logical knowledge is that which is used when a mathematical problem is solved, since the logical rules have been followed and a conclusion has been reached. Empirical knowledge is that which people gain through their senses. Pragmatic knowledge is experimental and individuals have it when they know that something they know actually works for them in practice – in this sense it is scientific. If that knowledge is not capable of producing the types of results that are expected, then it is rejected and new knowledge sought that works. Herein lies the idea of the human being as scientist, seeking always to understand and experiment upon social reality (Kelly, 1963). It should be noted that in the postmodern literature (for example, Lyotard, 1984) pragmatism is regarded as the sole legitimator of knowledge, reflecting the previous discussion which indicated the movement towards a greater emphasis on practice and less on theory.

However, this idea of experimentation is also quite crucial to understanding something of the relationship between personal knowledge and action – perhaps, between theory and practice. It is always a probability situation. Heller (1984 p166) suggests that the 'pragmatic relationship denotes the direct unity of theory and practice'. People almost always act upon the probability that the action will achieve the desired results, and they act with 'sufficient ground' (Heller, 1984 p169), that is to say that they have some knowledge that enables them to act in a certain way and that they believe that their action will have specific results, or else they will not so act. Pragmatic knowledge is a form of scientific knowledge that should underlie a great deal of all professional practitioners' actions. Because they know it works, it is necessarily conservative in nature – why should individuals change their behaviour when they know that what they are doing works? It is no good the theoretician trying to convince them that they are wrong, because they have proved to themselves that what they know works. However, they cannot necessarily control all the circumstances within which their actions occur, hence every situation is one of probability.

This is a weakness in Habermas' (1972) formulation of technical-cognitive knowledge. It will be recalled that Habermas also has three forms of knowledge or, as he calls them, processes of enquiry: the technical-cognitive, the historical-hermeneutic and the emancipatory. The technical cognitive form is about practical knowledge and he (1972 p309) regards this as having 'control over objectified processes'. Whilst this control may well refer to the human action itself, the possession of knowledge does not necessarily mean that those who possess it have control over the outcomes of the practical acts that stem from its utilization. It means only that they understand them.

It was Ryle who raised this question of practical knowledge in a seminal study in 1949. He (1963) distinguished between *knowledge how* and *knowledge that* and suggested that in everyday life 'we are more concerned with people's competences than with their cognitive repertoires' (1963 p28). Here he was attacking the intellectual emphasis upon cognitive knowledge, and yet he oversimplified the problem by adopting a behaviourist solution, and he suggested that when 'I am doing something intelligently . . . I am doing one thing and not two' (1963 p32). Here Ryle has actually confused three things: the skill, the knowledge how to perform the action, and the monitoring of the action. Ryle also implicitly raised two sets of inter-related problems: firstly, he implied that 'knowing how' and 'being able' are synonymous, which is incorrect; secondly, he demonstrates quite clearly that when people perform an action they cannot necessarily always articulate the theory underlying the action.

Sheffler (1965) also points out that *knowing how* and *being able* are not synonymous concepts. He provides the illustration of a person who might know how to drive a car but be prevented from doing so for a variety of reasons, for example, having a broken leg. There are contingencies that cannot always be controlled. The difference between having the knowledge and being able to perform the skill still remains crucial to this discussion. However, this illustration does not probe deeply enough and another question emerges – when people say 'I know how to . . .' are they really using a term that has a cognitive orientation at all? Would it not be more correct to claim that 'I am able to . . .'? In other words, the possession of a skill does not necessarily always mean that people have all, or much, of the *knowledge how*, although there may well be other occasions when they actually have or have had that knowledge. There are no doubt times when a skill is learned and only as it is being acquired do the actors gain any *knowledge how* and as they realize that there are alternative procedures that they might practise, they learn the *knowledge that* the different procedures will produce different outcomes, etc.

While Ryle's distinction between *knowing how* and *knowing that* is important, there is another dimension which he omitted – *knowing why* something is valid or not. Being able to understand why certain outcomes are likely to occur as a result of specific actions is a very important aspect of practical knowledge. Consequently, it might be argued that practical knowledge has at least three different forms of conscious knowledge. Practical knowledge is one element of theory – it is the theory *of* practice.

Having clarified the distinction between skill and elaborated on knowledge it is now possible to return to the idea of a field of practice and Figure 1.2 illustrates the inter-relationship between the practice and the practical knowledge that is required to perform the role.

It can be seen that all these three forms of knowledge are driven by practice. They are all pragmatic, in Sheffler's sense, and the expert practitioners have a considerable body of knowledge which relates to their

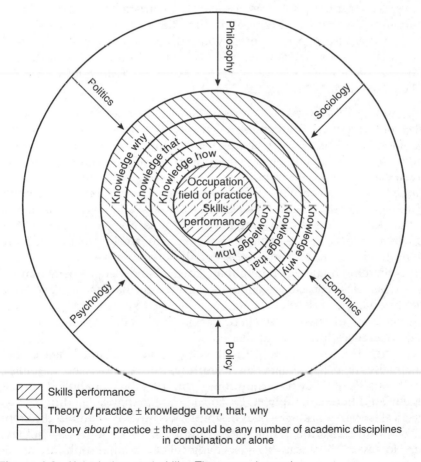

Skills performance

Theory *of* practice ± knowledge how, that, why

Theory *about* practice ± there could be any number of academic disciplines in combination or alone

Figure 1.2   Knowledge and skills: Theory and practice

own experience of practice, but there are occasions when they have habitualized their actions to such an extent that, even if they ever knew the underlying theory about certain aspects of their practice, they cannot specify precisely what it is. Additionally, they might also find it difficult to explain to others precisely how they perform certain procedures, etc. In a recent study about practical knowledge and expertise, Nyiri (1988 pp20–1) writes:

> One becomes an expert not simply by absorbing explicit knowledge of the type found in textbooks, but through experience, that is, through repeated trials, 'failing, succeeding, wasting time and effort . . . getting to feel the problem, learning to go by the book and when to break the rules'. Human experts thereby gradually absorb 'a repertory of working rules of thumb, or "heuristics", that, combined with book knowledge, make them expert practitioners'. This practical, heuristic knowledge, as attempts to simulate it on the machine have shown, is 'hardest to get at because experts – or anyone else – rarely have the self-awareness to recognize what it is. So it must be mined out of their heads painstakingly, one jewel at a time'. (All quotes from Feigenbaum and McCorduck, 1984)

Ryle may well be correct when he suggested that some of the original rules are forgotten through constant practice, but Nyiri is suggesting another element – that, through continuous experimentation, new knowledge is gradually absorbed from experience which might never have been articulated. Practical knowledge, then, is hidden in the practitioner, or as Polyani (1967) suggests, it has become tacit knowledge, i.e. knowledge that cannot necessarily be expressed in words. The nature of that knowledge is also pragmatic, i.e. it is accepted because it is known to work. But, because it is known to work, practitioners are loathe to change it, and so it is essentially conservative.

It is therefore maintained here that practical knowledge has two inter-related aspects: conscious cognitive knowledge, having at least three dimensions, and tacit knowledge. Learning tacit knowledge is a process that has been discussed elsewhere (Jarvis, 1994), although there will be more references to it later in this book.

The significant thing about this body of practical knowledge is that it is totally inter-disciplinary, there is no pure philosophy, no sociology, etc. It consists of its own constitution of different 'bits' of applied knowledge from different disciplines. Practical nursing knowledge differs from practical social work knowledge simply because it requires different skills and different mixes of applied philosophy, sociology, psychology, etc. However, there can be a sociological, or a philosophical, or an economic, etc. study of each field of practice but when the studies are located in the disciplines rather than in practice, they are driven by the internal logic of the discipline rather than the vicissitudes of practice. These studies constitute the second feature of theory: this is theory *about* practice.

The teacher practitioner and the mentor both exist to help the students, the new recruits or the junior colleagues to acquire some of this practical knowledge. Having begun to explore the nature of practical knowledge, it is now necessary to look at the role of the mentor.

THE MENTOR

Mentorship has suddenly assumed a respectability in professional education, and beyond, and those who use it often try to differentiate it from the image of the apprentice master, the teacher practitioner, etc. Indeed, there have been a number of attempts to define the term. Fish and Purr (1991 p47), for instance, say that 'nurses who supervize the clinical practice' are called mentors, and they briefly go on to highlight the relationship between the mentor and the student. Sloan and Slevin (1991 p20) suggest that, while there is no real agreement in the literature:

> as new entrants progress through the early experiences, they require considerable personal support (<u>mentorship</u>) and directive teaching-learning (<u>preceptorship</u>). Later they require more space, and the clinician's role is more of a <u>facilitator</u> – providing tuition at a more advanced level, being available on request, acting as a critic and a 'stimulator' of reflection in practice. (underlining in the original)

The passage then goes on to discuss yet another function, that of the role model. Obviously, these are all different functions in the teaching and learning process in practice and, if they were agreed upon as all being relevant, it would be possible for one, or more than one, person to perform the various functions stipulated here, and elsewhere. To have a variety of role players, however, as different occupational categories, would perhaps be excessive, so that these may merely reflect the different roles that one person might play. Such a person might be a teacher practitioner, a manager or a supervisor of professional practice – or even a mentor!

Both Fish and Purr and Sloan and Slevin seem to relate mentoring to professional practice only, whereas Carruthers (1993 p11) suggests that there is another form of mentoring which is as much concerned with personal development as with the professional development.

Defining the concept of mentor has run into several of the difficulties implicit in the above discussion, as Hagerty (1986) demonstrated when she claimed that the literature confuses the person, the process and the activities. But this is no less true of a word like 'teacher' and so the problems surrounding the concept of mentorship are not insurmountable, even though any resolution will not necessarily gain universal support. The concept of mentorship is now discussed, followed by an examination of the mentor's functions.

THE CONCEPT OF MENTORSHIP

There seems to be almost universal agreement that mentoring involves a relationship with the learner. Consequently, it is possible to begin to define the mentor relationship as *one in which two people relate to each other with the explicit purpose of the one assisting the other to learn.* The fact is that this relationship is explicitly a personal one-to-one relationship, and this is the crucial difference between the roles of mentor and teacher, although this does not necessarily apply in the case of the teacher practitioner; in mentoring the relationship comes closer to that of counsellors with those whom they counsel. However, the function of the relationship lies in mentors assisting the learners (or mentees, or protégés, to learn and to perform their role more effectively, or to develop themselves. Frequently, this may involve direct teaching although there are many occasions when the mentor is not the teacher, but may be a facilitator of reflective practice or an opener of doors that lead to other learning opportunities, etc. This concentration on the nature of a relationship appears to be another crucial difference between mentoring and teaching. However, it must be recognized that relationship lies at the heart of all social living and not something particular to the roles being discussed here.

Murray (1991 p5) points out that there are two schools of thought about mentoring: the one suggests that it can be structured or facilitated, while the other maintains that it can only happen when the 'chemistry' between the two people is right. However, these are not automatically exclusive, since a facilitated relationship might actually develop into one where the chemistry appears to be right for the relationship to continue and to deepen. Clearly, in education and training, structured or facilitated mentoring is called for and this creates a form of mentorship which is very similar to being a teacher practitioner but, unlike being a teacher practitioner, mentoring is not something that can just be turned on and off with the passing of every short module, etc. This has already been discovered in nursing when, as Barlow (1991) reports, short-term mentorship did not seem appropriate for clinical practice with students. Indeed, these mentors were often new staff nurses who would no doubt have benefitted from being mentored themselves. It is also for this reason that some branches of nursing have referred to this structured form of mentoring as preceptorship, which has been defined as 'a registered nurse who has been specially prepared to guide and direct student learning during clinical placements'.

It is the relationship which is important in mentoring – in Buber's (1959) words, it is an I–Thou relationship, and this is something which will be discussed more fully in Chapter 2.

But who is the mentor? On occasions the mentor can be the teacher, but on others the mentor may be an adviser, a senior colleague or an expert. Occasionally, it can be the manager – but it might be difficult to enter such a relationship with an immediately junior colleague, so that where there is a facilitated mentor relationship the mentor is often at least two rungs higher than the protégé.

THE FUNCTIONS OF THE MENTOR

It is clear from this discussion that mentoring is not regarded here in the same light as coaching (Schon, 1987) or supervising in clinical practice, or even personal tutoring (Barlow, 1991). However, there is a sense in which the personal tutor can become a mentor with students, as Daloz (1986) demonstrates in liberal adult education where adults are returning to college to study. But if the mentor is to play a role in education and the professions, especially after the mentee has graduated, then the personal tutor may not be able to perform it and, in some cases, the ex-students may not want it. Hence, it seems that Murray's (1991) distinction between facilitated and unstructured mentoring becomes even more important. During studentship, some form of mentor role might be performed by the personal tutor, especially one who is acknowledged to be concerned about excellence in practice. Mentorship might also be facilitated for junior qualified staff, in the way that Murray indicates. She (1991 p58) records a top level executive as saying:

'I'm always mentoring, both formally and informally. My role is to help my subordinates make decisions. I let them bounce ideas off me and I give my input. But ultimately, I want them to make decisions. If I were making all the decisions for them, I wouldn't need them, would I? So taking on what you call an "additional protégé" is no great hardship for me in terms of time. It's what I do anyway.'

Here the distinction between acting formally and informally is important – perhaps the informal mentoring relationship, which just emerges or emerges after the formal relationship has been created, is at the heart of mentoring.

In his excellent book on mentoring, Daloz (1986 pp215–35) suggests some of the major things that good mentors do in the situations of mentoring adult students, and he does so under three headings – support, challenge and provide a vision. Each of these are sub-divided into a number of different functions:

- *Support* – listening, providing structure, expressing positive expectations, sharing ourselves, making it special
- *Challenge* – setting tasks, engaging in discussion, heating up dichotomies, constructing hypotheses, setting high standards
- *Vision* – modelling, keeping tradition, offering a map, suggesting new language, providing a mirror.

Morton-Cooper and Palmer (1993 pp62–4) also suggest a number of different functions of the mentor; they specify eight: adviser; coach, counsellor; guide/networker; role model; sponsor; teacher; resource facilitator.

In a sense, in these instances, the role of the mentor is to help the protégés to reflect on their practice, to learn from their experiences and to improve their practice and to develop themselves, so that they might exercise even more expertise and maturity. In mentoring, this is done through an in-depth relationship whether it is structured or informal, a primary experience, Buber's educative relationship. Indeed, it is the relationship that makes mentorship so important – not just to professional practice. It is then not only in practice that the mentee gains, it is also a life-enriching relationship – but should the mentor also gain from such a relationship?

> But connections achieve ... only in so far as they make the existence of the connected into *being for each other*, not merely being *with* each other. My continued being 'makes sense' only in as far as there are others who go on needing me. Beckoning to me, making me attentive to their plight, filling me with the feeling of responsibility for them, they make me unique, irreplaceable, indispensable individual that I am: the entity whose disappearance would make a hole in the universe, create that void ... Unless 'I am *for*, I am not. (Bauman, 1992a p40)

Being open to others is at the heart of human being, but if the mentor smothers the mentee, then the fears expressed by Burnard are justified. Mentorship is about exercising this human characteristic in genuine dialogue, so that ultimately both develop and feel needed through the relationship.

THE TEACHER

Malcolm Knowles (1980 p26) claims that many people perform a teaching role and, indeed, they do. However, they do not all have to be teacher trained in order to teach, since anybody who facilitates another's learning may be regarded as an educator. Mentors may be more rarely trained for mentoring but they might certainly be regarded as teachers or facilitators of others' learning. Even so, in the case of the teacher practitioner, the role is much more specific, since it involves inducting the student into the work situation, which may be located in a ward, a community setting, a department in a school or college, etc. Yet it is more than merely a process of induction, it is an active teaching role in an interpersonal situation. Two points arise from this – they are both roles of educators of adults (although mentoring can occur with children) and they are of an interpersonal nature.

There is an increasingly significant body of knowledge emerging about the art of teaching adults and a considerable amount of research results are beginning to appear about individualized learning, so that it is important for teacher practitioners and mentors to be aware of this work. Unfortunately, the body of literature on the art and science of teaching adults in an interpersonal, one-to-one situation is still small although it is growing (for example, Megginson and Clutterbuck, 1995).

While mentors and teacher practitioners may not always regard themselves as teachers of adults and may not regard their occupation as adult educators, they actually straddle the expertise of two professions – their own and that of educators of adults. But the concept of profession has never been agreed upon by scholars and so it is wiser here to separate occupational structures (profession) from occupational attitudes (professionalism), and it is much more significant to enquire whether teacher practitioners are professional teachers than to ask whether they are members of two professions. The teacher practitioners should be experts in teaching adults in an interpersonal situation; they should have both the knowledge and skill to undertake this role with competence. Additionally, since the body of knowledge in the education of adults is expanding rapidly, they should be endeavouring to keep abreast with all of these developments, so that they can offer their learners the most expert service. Hence, teacher practitioners should be both professional teachers and professional practitioners in order to perform their role: this combination of professionalisms is the essence of their role.

Such an argument also holds good for those mentors who facilitate and structure learning, whose role is *de facto* that of teacher practitioner even though they may be called mentors. Those unstructured mentoring situations which exist because of the relationship, much more than because of the expertise of the mentor, are discussed more fully in Chapter 2.

STRADDLING TWO PROFESSIONALISMS

The teacher practitioner and those mentors are, therefore, in a most interesting position, they straddle two professionalisms and should be experts in both. Such a role has its own responsibilities, rewards and problems. They should keep abreast of new knowledge and skills in their practice, but at the same time they are required to be aware of new educational knowledge and to be skilful in the manner by which they facilitate the learning of their students. But there is only a limited amount of time for reading and studying, and few people are prepared or are able to devote all their leisure (if they have any!) to work preparation, so that they are frequently confronted with a dilemma – wherein do they place their energies? This problem is exacerbated when they have heavy workloads, as is increasingly happening in the Health and Social Services, since they are still expected to continue their professional practice as well as to teach the learners. In the ward situation, it might sometimes be possible for the clinical nurse having a teaching role to assume it quite specifically for some time, whilst colleagues concentrate more on their clinical roles. But this type of division of labour cannot occur so easily in the community where, for instance, practice teachers are independent professional practitioners. Students may, therefore, be viewed as additional burdens to an already overloaded practice.

Straddling two professional roles has, however, a great many rewards as well as additional responsibilities: it can, for instance, result in job satisfaction at two levels, that of caring for patients/clients and that of helping students and junior colleagues to improve their own practice. This latter aspect has the additional bonus of knowing that the teacher practitioners' own standards of role performance can be maintained and perpetuated, in part, since they can learn from their students and junior colleagues as well as teach them. Yet it must be recognized that, however rewarding the work, straddling two professional roles is both a difficult and demanding task for those who undertake it and it is one that teacher practitioners will inevitably perform in different ways.

Some teacher practitioners may discover that they prefer professional practice and get more satisfaction from its performance, others may find more pleasure from conducting their teaching role and assisting learners to become more competent practitioners, while a third group may gain satisfaction from combining both teaching and practising. Some teacher practitioners might ultimately resign from their teaching role in order to concentrate on professional practice. Many others, for example, ward managers, have little choice and are required to perform both of these roles, plus their managerial one. However, if teacher practitioners and occasionally nurse teachers are available to assist ward managers, some of the latter may find great satisfaction in mentoring, etc.

The teacher practitioner's role straddles two entirely different professionalisms, yet it is a specific role. It is, in many ways, amongst the most significant in any occupation since it combines theory, practice and the teaching of practice. Nursing and to some extent social work, unlike many professions, have recognized the importance of the role and have offered some form of preparation for it. The teacher practitioner's role is not only highly skilled but also very significant because it lies at the interfaces of theory and practice and occupational preparation and practice.

THE TEACHER PRACTITIONER WITHIN PROFESSIONAL EDUCATION AND TRAINING

Teacher practitioners are practitioners and so they are also teachers of professional skills. Their own professional experience means that they have built up their own repertoire of expertise, but they have to be aware that they do not assume their expertise in such a way that they cannot teach it. What should make them different from the expert discussed earlier is that they are aware of the way that skills are performed and are able to teach learners how to perform them.

In students' minds it is easy for theory and practice to become divorced: it is quite common to hear learners, returning to a school or college after a period of professional practical experience, exclaim how much they had enjoyed their practice but how irrelevant the theoretical knowledge appears. A variety of reasons may exist for this, including:

- Practice is obviously very relevant to what the students are looking for and so theory seems distant from it.
- Theory tends to be abstract, generalized and impersonal whereas practice appears concrete, specific and personal.
- Theory is sometimes taught in an uninteresting fashion and not applied to the actual occupational experience.
- Teachers of theory may be far removed from practice and immersed in it for its own sake.
- Modular systems of training may not be in operation and the theory may not be immediately applicable to the students' current work situation.
- The theory taught is discipline-based rather than practice-based and, while it is necessary to have some discipline-based understanding, it is more important to have a good grasp of practical knowledge from the outset.

- Teachers might come from the disciplines rather than from practice, and this is increasingly likely as nursing and social work education becomes more closely integrated into higher education.

None of these reasons is an excuse for poor teaching but they are offered as examples of reasons why students may feel that the two are so far apart.

Yet a great deal of curriculum knowledge, i.e. theoretical knowledge, is included in the curriculum by the different professions's ruling bodies. However, there is often a lack of sophisticated understanding between the two types of theory – theory *of* practice and theory *about* practice, the former being practice-driven and the latter driven from the demands of the cognate disciplines themselves. It is important that this difference is fully recognized in curriculum planning. It is at this interface of practice and practical knowledge that the teacher practitioners and mentors perform much of their roles. It is not just a matter of helping the students and the new entrants to the profession to utilize the practical knowledge that they have been taught, it is also a matter of helping them become reflective practitioners and to learn from their own practice so that they can begin to construct and enlarge their own bodies of practical knowledge.

Teaching theory has often been equated with 'education' while the teaching of practical skills has usually been called 'training'. Education has been regarded as a high status process and training as low status. However, with the emergence of the idea of practical knowledge, this distinction is becoming blurred, and it has been argued elsewhere (Jarvis, 1983a; Pring, 1993) that this distinction is over-simplistic and that training may also be educational. Indeed, with the growth of the idea of continuing education, and the development of such new degree courses as practitioner doctorates, this crude separation between education and training should be regarded as something historical and, especially in vocational education, the two should be combined since practice and practical knowledge are pragmatically related and cannot be separated.

The preparation of professionals should always be regarded as an educational process, even when they are learning skills. However, there are sociological studies that examine the reasons why theoretical knowledge has high status and practical knowledge has low status (for example, Young, 1971), and the fact that this actually occurs does mean that teacher practitioners, despite their very significant role, usually have lower status than the lecturer of theory in higher education. At the same time, their role is significant in professional preparation and, as was pointed out earlier, they often become role models for the new recruits to the profession. In addition, they are most frequently the assessors of students' performances so that they also become the gate-keepers to the profession; assessment is a subject to which further reference is made later in the book and so it will not be discussed further here.

Teacher practitioners and mentors, therefore, occupy a significant place in the preparation and development of recruits to, and junior staff in, the profession: without such roles the education, training and professional and personal development of students and staff would be impoverished beyond measure.

Conclusion

This chapter has examined the roles of the mentor and the teacher practitioner, highlighting some of its significant features and illustrating some of its satisfaction and challenges. Their role is of a dual nature, practising and teaching, in which there are inherent conflicts and tremendous opportunities. However, the concern of this book is the performance of the educational and developmental elements of the roles and so the focus of the remainder of the book is on these processes, rather than the actual professional performance of the practitioners. Consequently, Chapter 2 focuses upon the teaching and learning transaction, in which the interaction between the teachers/facilitators and the learners is examined.

Teaching, mentoring and the learning interaction

2

This chapter explores:
- *The teacher–learner relationship*
- *Interpersonal skills*
- *The roles of the teacher and mentor.*

INTRODUCTION

Often the process of teaching and learning is referred to as a transaction, but it is suggested here that it is more appropriate to regard it as an interaction (Jarvis, 1995b) rather than a transaction, since the former term has connotations of a business exchange. At the same time, it is recognized that teaching and learning, when adults and professionals are concerned, involves negotiation since the teacher does not know everything. The idea that the teacher knows everything is a very traditional and authoritarian view of education, one that no doubt reflects the experience of many adults in their initial education and even, perhaps, in their professional preparation. Yet this approach is foreign to the ethos of the education of adults, especially in an individualized teaching and learning situations of mentoring and preceptorship, etc.

Perhaps education itself should always involve negotiation between teacher and learner, but much more in the sense of interaction than business transaction, even though the status of the teacher in primary education is rather different from that of the five-year-olds whom she teaches. Education might be defined as 'any planned series of incidents, having a humanistic basis, directed towards the participant(s) learning and understanding' (Jarvis 1983a p5). This definition presupposes that the humanity of the participant(s) is paramount in the educational process, so that when there is only one teacher and one learner involved it is hardly surprising that considerable emphasis should be placed upon the interpersonal interaction in the teaching and learning process.

Over two decades ago, Kidd (1973 p269) suggested that there are five fundamental elements in most teaching and learning transactions:

- the learner
- the teacher
- the group
- the setting or situation
- the subject matter.

As education is changing, some of these five are no longer essential elements since, for instance, there might not be a single teacher in distance education. In addition, in individualized teaching and learning, the group is not present, as Kidd himself recognized. However, there may be occasions when the teacher practitioner has more than one student and while she is instructing one of them, she realizes that it would be useful for other learners to join in the learning process, so that she then creates a small group.

The setting, or situation, is a significant element in the interaction that takes place in individualized teaching and learning and mentoring, but it is a feature infrequently mentioned in many textbooks on education because it is automatically assumed that the setting for teaching and learning is the classroom. Some books concerned with the education of adults (for example, Rogers, 1977 pp101–5; 1989 pp83–6) concentrate on the arrangements of furniture in the classroom, suggesting that the desks or tables, etc. should be arranged in circles in order to facilitate discussion amongst learners.

However, as there is now more concern about learning in the workplace, there is a greater recognition about the various potential learning situations. In individualized teaching and learning there may be no classroom teaching, so that the choice of the situation remains with the participants. Often it is the responsibility of the teacher practitioner to decide when the situation is appropriate to raise an issue, but sometimes the learner might wish to question the teacher, so that in this instance it is the learner's responsibility to choose the setting for the interaction to occur. However, when the teacher makes the choice, great care should be given to making a selection in order to ensure that it is most suited for the teaching and learning to occur. The choice may actually involve the teacher practitioner preparing the setting beforehand, but this might not always be necessary, possible or appropriate. Some of the situations in which the teaching and learning interaction might occur are listed in Table 2.1.

Clearly some of these locations are rather public and the discretion of the teacher practitioner must be used in all circumstances. In addition, some of the venues may be rather exposed to other people overhearing the teaching and learning transaction, which might not be appropriate.

Table 2.1 Some possible teaching and learning situations

For the ward manager, clinical teacher or nurse/midwife teacher in an institution	For teacher practitioner in the community
Ward/department/theatre	Health centre office
Manager's/charge nurse's office	Health centre treatment room
Interview room	Interview room
Hospital corridors	Health centre staff room
Staff room	House of client/patient
Staff canteen	Car (teacher's or student's)
Seminar/Tutorial room	Staff canteen

Obviously one of the most frequent places where this form of individualized teaching and mentoring takes place is in the public view of the patients, clients, relatives and staff. Care must be taken to ensure that there is a genuinely human interaction when this occurs in public view so that the learner's self image is in no way threatened by such a public exposure. It might also be considered impolite to teach a student in the presence of the patient/client, unless the latter has agreed that it should happen, so that the teacher practitioner or mentor should always ensure that the patient/client in no way feels threatened by the situation. When teaching in public view, confidentiality must never be compromised.

All teacher practitioners are aware of their own work situation, so that they should be cognisant of the possibilities that exist and be prepared to utilize them in an appropriate manner. Some teacher practitioners have been able to negotiate the use of a room in close proximity to their clinical work situation which they can utilize for teaching purposes. This is obviously an ideal situation which enables the teaching and learning to proceed with less disturbance. However, it may be inferred from Table 2.1 that the teaching and learning interaction may not always be formalized, ideal or institutional in nature. However, the location of the teaching and learning is of lesser importance than the climate set for the interaction. Heath (1979) described an appropriate learning climate as one in which 'the learner can take risks (in the sense of trying out new behaviours), admit to difficulties and problems, give and receive feedback and cope with allied stress' (cited from Alexander, 1983 p41).

Of the remaining items from Kidd's five elements: the content will be discussed in Chapter 3 on designing a learning programme, and human learning is considered in Chapter 4, so that the teaching element alone remains for elaboration here. It is clear from this initial discussion that individualized teaching and learning relies heavily upon human interaction and a prerequisite for its success lies in the establishment of an effective working relationship between the teacher practitioner and the learner.

THE TEACHER–LEARNER RELATIONSHIP

The traditional image of the teacher standing before a class of students expounding the mysteries of knowledge about which the teacher is an expert is hardly appropriate to the forms of teaching and learning being discussed here. Neither are the conventional images of the student sitting at the feet of the guru awaiting with patience to receive the pearls of wisdom that he is prepared to cast forth, or of the apprentice looking over the master's shoulder watching the expert at work and thereby hoping to acquire sufficient knowledge to emulate his feats or expertise. Even so, it is recognized that there is a place for the demonstration of skills in the interpersonal teaching and learning situation in which the teacher practitioner or the mentor participate, but it may not be as significant as some people assume. Nevertheless, this approach is still predominant in some professional spheres but where it occurs it may be regarded as rather anachronistic, reflecting an approach that assumes that the experts can pass on their skills effectively to the student, simply because they are expert practitioners. Little concern is paid in either of these conventional approaches to the skills of teaching or to the relationship of the teacher with the student. Explicit to this discussion is an emphasis on the inter-personal aspects of the relationship, in which the dignity and humanity of both participants are fully recognized and respected.

Even so, it might be argued that the dignity and the humanity of the participants may still be respected in a hierarchical relationship, with the teacher practitioner exercising the authority of her position over the learners. Radical educators (for example, Bowles and Gintis, 1976) have claimed that education tends to prepare learners to accept hierarchical relationships in the work situation because teaching and learning is conducted within a hierarchical context. While Bowles and Gintis referred to the school and to the education of children, it might be argued that similar processes still occur in education at most levels, despite the efforts of many educators to change their approach. The process that occurs is part of what some scholars regard as the hidden curriculum, a concept that will be discussed below, but it is clear that through such a curriculum education does tend to be reproductive, despite all the efforts of many educators.

Nevertheless, this hierarchical relationship is not one which should be reproduced in the individualized, non-formal teaching and learning situation within which much of the teacher practitioner's and mentor's teaching should be conducted. However, it might be realistic to claim that since the majority of learners are prepared for employment in the Health and Social Services, which have hierarchical structures, they should be prepared within one. Yet the aims of professional education (see Jarvis 1983a pp31–49) do not include reproducing the social hierarchy of the employing organization, but rather producing individuals who can think and act independently and critically in both a work and non-work situation. Hence, the hierarchical approach should be eschewed in individualized teaching and learning, indeed it should seldom be included in any form of education, especially in the education of adults.

Hence, it may be asked, what authority does the teacher practitioner possess, since teacher practitioners usually occupy higher positions in the Health Service hierarchy than do their learners? For instance, the ward manager is responsible for the smooth organization of the ward and the standard of nursing care given to the patients within it, while the learners may be accountable to her in part for the care that they render patients. Note, however, that this accountability is for the performance of the nursing role. At the same time the ward manager might well set learning objectives for her staff and then the staff on the ward are accountable to the manager for their learning as well. Although the ward manager's authority is that of ward manager rather than that of teacher practitioner; she should gain the respect of her learners because of her knowledge and skill. Similarly, if a community practice teacher were teaching a senior nurse manager about some technique developed in the community, she would have no authority over the manager, yet she should still command the respect of the senior nurse manager because of her knowledge and skill. The authority of the teacher practitioner is that granted to her by the learners who respect her professionalism. But if she cannot gain that respect, then the teacher practitioner has no authority, as teacher, in the eyes of the learners. Professional authority finds its legitimation in the recognition given to the practitioner by peers, clients and students, but not in the position occupied in the hierarchy. Hence, the authority of the teacher practitioner resides entirely in the recognition of her professionalism, and that of the mentor because the mentee grants it. At the same time, it must be recognized that many learners do look for role models in people who have status in the profession (Fretwell, 1982, Melia, 1983), although their professional – but not their bureaucratic – authority can soon disappear if high status people are found to be bad practitioners!

Yet learners also bring to the teaching and learning interaction their own ideas and experiences, the results of their reading and study, thoughts about new techniques, etc. that they have learned in school, college or professional practice, so that the teacher has also opportunity to learn from the learner. But if there is no genuine relationship as such, interchange might not occur and then the teacher practitioner would not benefit from the student, and as a result she would be intellectually impoverished. It will, no doubt, have been noted that in the definition of education cited earlier in this chapter there was reference to the participants' learning, but no reference to the teacher. Additionally, in Kidd's five points, the teacher's place was queried. Teachers are not essential to education, but learners are! Teachers are, however, very useful adjuncts to the educational process, but the richer the interchange between teacher and learner, and learner and teacher, the more both participants are likely to learn. Freire (1972a p53) claimed that a teacher–student relationship is contrary to the dialogical relationship that should emerge in problem-solving learning and he suggested that the relationship should be regarded as a teacher/student–student/teacher one, in which both participants engage in both roles to their mutual benefit. This is interaction, rather than transaction, that has been discussed already in this book.

Perhaps the crucial idea in teaching and learning lies in the word 'relationship'. Teaching and learning in the individualized situation, although not in all forms of distance education, involves a unique relationship between the teacher, or mentor, and the learner and, consequently, it is with the work of some philosophers who have concentrated their analyses on 'relationship' that this part of the discussion turns. Of these, perhaps the most well-known in adult education is Martin Buber, although there are many other eminent philosophers whose work is important to this discussion.

Buber, in a number of major works, explored the idea of relationship, especially in *I and Thou* (1959) and *Between Man and Man* (1947). In *I and Thou* he explored the idea of personal relationship, as opposed to I–It relationships. He might also have, but did not, postulate a third form of relationship, I–Group relationship, since there are many occasions, especially in education, where individuals are confronted with a group, or an agglomeration of individuals. While such interaction might be regarded as impersonal, it is not the same as trying to interact with a tree, so that it must be seen as a form of personal relationship.

For Buber, the personal relationship is conducted at three levels – with living being, with individual persons and with spiritual beings – each of which could be expanded upon here, but only the second of these is relevant to the present discussion. People enter personal relationships through direct experience, usually because they share the same space at the same time and through so doing they have opportunity to interact with each other during which time they share a mutual bond. Before a relationship is formed, I exist in my world and the Other is a stranger, a significant idea since the stranger is free (Levinas, 1991 p39) over whom I have no power. When I enter relationship with the Other, especially if the Other is an adult, it is usually through the medium of language in the first instance, although relationship is more than an exchange of words. When I and the Other are face-to-face, the distance between the Stranger and me recedes and some form of bond begins to be created, but the very formation of that bond impinges upon the freedom which is the prerogative of the Other. At the same time, my own freedom in respect to the Other is curtailed. The bond's existence, however weak, signifies that I am prepared to forego some of my freedom in order to enter a relationship. This relationship may be only for a brief period of time, although there is potentiality for it to continue beyond the first interaction.

I am able to enter such a relationship with the Other for whatever period of time it exists because of our common humanity. Where there is no humanity, the relationship is of necessity an I–It one. Relationships with a group, because all its members are human beings, share many of the same characteristics as with the Other, but they tend to develop the bonds of community rather than those of the more exclusive personal relationship. (The exclusive personal relationship always puts the community at risk, since it has the power to fragment the group.) The potentiality of individual personal relationships always exists in the educational situation. Herein lies a fundamental truth, when the I–Thou relationship is formed the Stranger, or the group member, becomes a person with whom I, as a person, can share a human bond. My personhood can only be realized in relationship with another person – or as Buber (1959 p18) put it, 'In the beginning is relationship', and MacMurray (1961 p17) suggested 'the Self is constituted by its relation to the Other'. Elsewhere, MacMurray (1961 p24) claimed that 'the idea of an isolated Agent is self-contradictory. Any Agent is necessarily is relation to Other. Apart from this essential relationship he [sic] does not exist'.

As the relationship becomes established, certain patterns of interaction begin to appear and it is these which curtail freedom. Sociologists call these norms and mores, and some scholars (such as Heller, 1988) wrongly regard these as the foundation of ethics, although it must be recognized that values, both moral and immoral, are manifest within norms and mores. Like the case studies, norms may not reflect the morality of the interaction for a number of reasons, including the fact that the norms of modernity were shown above to be morally flawed in certain situations. Additionally, if there is an unequal power between the actors, the patterns of interaction may reflect the selfish desires of the more powerful actor even though they may not be presented to the less powerful or even to the general public, in this manner. This is a danger that those who act as teachers and mentors frequently face. Hence, it appears that the actual location of morality lies with the intention of the actors rather than with the behaviour itself. One of the problems with this is that individuals can claim that they had good intentions, even though their actions had unfortunate outcomes and, in other situations, bad intentions can produce a good outcome – but in these latter situations the morality underlying the action has to be questioned. Consequently, ethics is not an empirical science! It is grounded in human intention, wherein the morality of action lies.

It is in a common humanity that the foundations of arguments for ethics lies and in the formation of the relationship in which personhood may be realized rests the practicalities of ethics. Indeed, Levinas (1991 p43) argues that ethics arise when an individual's spontaneity is inhibited by the presence of Other, and if this position is accepted then teaching must always be seen to be an occupation grounded in the moral debate. (He actually regards the bond that is established between the Self and the Other, the I–Thou relationship, as religion, and MacMurray develops his discussion in a similar manner with a discussion of the celebration of communion, although this point will not be developed further here.) However, it is clear that in the potentiality of personal relationship itself lies the basis of any discussion of the nature of ethical value. MacMurray (1961 p116) would agree with this analysis and he claimed that the 'moral rightness of an action . . . has its grounds in the relation of persons'.

It is significant that whatever the relationship, whoever the people and whatever the historical time, this argument still applies. It is for these reasons that it can be claimed that the basis of moral value is that it is universalizable, i.e. applied to every situation. It may thus be seen why Kant claimed that values had to be generalizable in this manner, which is implicit in MacMurray's (1961 p122) claim that:

> To act rightly is . . . to act for the sake of the Other and not of oneself. The Other . . . always remains fully personal; consequently its objectives must be the maintaining of positive personal relations between all agents as the bond of community.

The underlying point here is that the intention behind the action is some form of care, or concern, for the Other. It is maintained that such an intention is never wrong in itself, except when the desire to care for one Other may put many others at risk, and this illustrates the distinction between the I–Thou and the I–Group relationship. Clearly in this instance, there is a major ethical debate about putting one's loved ones before unknown Others, or the teacher devoting more effort to favoured learners than to the class as a whole. Teachers must be concerned for all those with whom they work and act for their own sake rather than the teachers' own self-interest. At the same time teachers interact with all the class individually, so that there is both an I–Group interaction and a potential I–Thou relationship with each individual member of the class. Since these are both personal in nature, the I–Thou relationship will constitute the basis of the following analysis and its significance for the I–Group relationship will be discussed in the conclusion.

In individualized teaching and learning, this would appear to be the most appropriate form of relationship, and the only one which has a genuinely moral basis. It is one for which teacher practitioners and mentors should strive to gain with their students and mentees. However, it is recognized that it is one which might be difficult to achieve because of the hierarchical nature of the work situation. Such a relationship depends on the personal skills of the participants.

INTERPERSONAL SKILLS

It will be apparent from the foregoing discussion that the creation of a relationship of trust and respect is an essential precursor to an enriching teaching and learning transaction. While there is always responsibility on both participants to form such a bond, it must be recognized that the initiative for this lies with teachers and mentors. Hence, it is essential from the outset for them to recognize that their role is not merely that of communicating knowledge and skills to the learners, but of creating an environment in which the teaching and learning interaction can be enriched to their mutual benefit. Research conducted in the late 1970s and early 1980s demonstrates that the attainment of such an environment is not easy in a busy ward, unless staff, teachers and students are mutually supportive (Fretwell, 1979; Ogier, 1982; Orton, 1981; Alexander, 1983; *et al.*).

Much has been written about interpersonal skills and it would perhaps be unwise to devote too great a space to repeating it here. Nevertheless, it is essential for the teacher practitioners or the mentors to have self-awareness and to have sufficient self-confidence to step out from behind the barriers of their organizational authority in order to try to create the type of relationship in which the learners can feel free to be themselves. This is an extremely difficult undertaking for some people, in the first instance, but the more that the teacher practitioners and mentors empathize with the learners and seek to understand the latters' own perception of themselves (including their own self-confidence and self-esteem), the greater the chance of creating such an environment. In short, the teacher practitioner and the mentor need to be self-confident and sensitive if they are to create a supportive relationship in which the learners have the opportunity to develop as independent thinkers and practitioners.

The teachers and mentors should, therefore, spend some time getting to know, on both a personal and a professional level, the students or mentees with whom they are working, and this may be done before they read any previous reports about the learners. Student notes are apt to influence the reader and to label the students or mentees for the teacher practitioners and mentors before the latter see them perform. It is the responsibility of the teacher practitioners and mentors 'to break the ice' with the students in an individualized teaching and learning situation and this may best be done in an informal situation, even away from the work environment if that is possible. Time is always a problem and rarely do the teacher practitioners or mentors have the time, so that an initial meeting may have to occur over a shared coffee break, etc.

However, some institutions now incorporate the initial informal contact between teacher practitioner and learner into the formalized part of the course; this practice is to be encouraged. But wherever it occurs, the first meeting is very important. In a slightly different context, and yet a very similar manner, adult educators recognize the importance of creating the right atmosphere in their class from the outset, so that their preparation for the first meeting may be even more rigorous than that for the classes that they conduct thereafter. The climate created in the first meeting will affect the remainder of the teaching and learning process, so that teacher practitioners should recognize that the student may:

- be rather anxious and need some reassurance
- have questions about the teaching and learning situation but not the confidence to ask them
- want to know the type of situation in which she will be working, for example, practice, regulations
- want to know some of the expectations that the teacher practitioner has of her
- want to be told about the teaching and learning programme.

Hence, the teacher practitioners should ensure that, from the outset, they invite the student to ask questions and make certain that adequate time is allowed at their first encounter to answer these in an unhurried and interested manner. Additionally, the teacher practitioners may anticipate certain questions and prepare a handout for reference purposes, which they can leave with the learners at the end of the first discussion. But during the meeting itself the learners might generally be encouraged to talk, ask questions and generally feel at ease in the interaction. Additionally, they should be invited to feel free to seek further clarification on anything that occurs during the teaching and learning interaction at any time.

Training in interpersonal skills in order to undertake the teacher practitioner role does not always occur in the short courses that are mounted as preparation for this role, even though it may be mentioned in the suggested curriculum. Kitchen (1993 p102) claims that preceptor training is a priority commitment in establishing a successful training programme in a hospital. Rarely are mentors trained in this way at all, although Walker and Stott (1993 pp74–90) record how school principals are prepared in Singapore through a mentoring scheme, in which the mentors are trained and developed as the scheme progresses. In addition, Carter (1993) suggests that trainers should be coached to perform their role in the workplace and he outlines a process that might usefully be employed. Indeed, the United Kingdom Central Council for Nursing, Midwifery and Health Visiting has stated quite specifically that preceptors should be prepared for their work, although it suggests that such preparation might be carried out over as short a period as two days (UKCC, 1993).

Teacher practitioners and mentors must be aware of the importance of these skills and seek consciously to develop them in their daily work with both their students and mentees and, significantly, with each other. It is important that those performing the teacher practitioner and mentoring roles are given opportunity to share their experiences with each other in order to learn from each other. The work environment certainly lends itself to this type of development, since teacher practitioners and mentors are always involved in relationships with their clients, patients, students and peers. The acquisition of the following skills may prove useful for the teacher practitioner:

- listening
- hearing what is said and noting what is left unsaid
- detecting emotional signals
- noting other non-verbal cues
- responding appropriately in a caring manner.

Teacher practitioners may consider that these are the skills of a sensitive person and ones that should be exercised by any social worker, nurse, midwife or health visitor. This is true, since they are the skills upon which the practice of the caring professions are based and it must be recognized that teaching is also a caring profession, so that these skills must be applied quite deliberately in an individualized teaching and learning or mentoring interaction. In addition, teacher practitioners should spend time reflecting on the process of teaching and learning in order to ensure that their skills are highly developed.

Individualized teaching and learning in a non-formal environment clearly raises questions about the roles that the teacher practitioners and mentors perform since it is clear that they are not merely the persons who transmit knowledge and skills for the student to acquire.

THE ROLES OF THE TEACHER AND MENTOR

The role of the mentor was explored in Chapter 1 and so the focus here is upon the actual teaching roles in the teaching and learning interaction. Once a personal relationship has been established between the teacher, or mentor, and the student, the former is exposed to the possibility of playing more parts than just that of the fount of wisdom and the clinical specialist; she may gain the roles of academic adviser, sympathetic listener and counsellor.

While this is not often the teacher practitioners' designated responsibility, since it is quite common for students to have a personal tutor and some colleges also employ the services of a professional counsellor, they are roles that are often played by them and it is difficult not to fulfil these without putting the interpersonal relationship at risk. As academic adviser, the teacher practitioner may be asked by the student: about aspects of the course theory being studied; for help with her coursework assignments; about the relationship between theory and practice. As a counsellor, the teacher practitioner may be exposed to some of the problems that the student is experiencing on the course, or even in her personal life. Teacher practitioners should not be expected to be fully trained counsellors, but it is useful to have a minimum of counselling skills to help the student explore the situation so that she can make her own informed decision. They should also have sufficient knowledge to be able to distinguish between the problems experienced by the student which are no more than the normal stresses, strains and crises of confidence that students sometimes experience during a course of study and those that require expert help. However well qualified in counselling the teacher practitioner may be, if she is to concentrate on her teaching role she may wish to refer any student requiring such assistance to the professional student counsellor employed by the educational institution, if such a service is available.

Some of these arguments also apply to the mentoring role, but since this is often informal and unstructured, there are fewer parameters that define the role. Mentors may well be asked to perform a wide range of roles, some of which will almost certainly involve counselling and support. The extent to which they feel that they can play these additional roles is an important consideration within the relationship, and they would be unwise to endeavour to play roles for which they have had no preparation or have little expertise.

Teacher practitioners, or mentors, who establish a good relationship with the learners or mentees may well become their confidante. Being entrusted with confidences is a responsibility that they should expect, value and respond to in the same manner in which they were shared. Hence, they should not break any confidence that they are given and if they consider something which they have been told should be revealed to others in the work environment, or the college or university, they should first seek permission from the mentee or student concerned to reveal it. Breaking confidence might destroy the relationship that they have endeavoured to establish and, however hard they then try to re-establish it, they will probably not be trusted again by the student, so that it is also doubtful whether they would then be able to fulfil their role effectively. It might be asked whether there are any times when such confidences might be broken – for instance, when a student might be suicidal – and the only response one can make is that there are ultimately no rules in moral interaction except being concerned for the Other. Consequently, the moral agent has to decide for herself what she considers best for the Other and act accordingly.

Not only do teachers and mentors perform these personal roles, they also perform a variety of teaching roles. Kidd (1973 p293) suggests that these include:

- animating and inspiring attention and commitment
- presenting information or demonstrating processes*
- raising relevant questions, developing habits of self-questioning*
- clarifying difficulties or obscurities*
- drawing parallels or finding relationships
- reflecting feelings
- expressing agreement and support
- evaluating, or developing the learner's capacity for self-evaluation*
- facilitating contacts+
- providing advice and guidance+.

Of these ten points the four marked with an asterisk will be developed in detail elsewhere, the final two, marked with +, are additions made by the authors, but included within the six which are discussed below.

ANIMATING

Most people who embark upon preparation for a profession are highly committed to the idea of entry to that occupation, so that at one level, seeking to inspire commitment is unnecessary. But at another level, in endeavouring to inspire the new entrant or the mentee to keep abreast with the developments in the theory and practice of the occupation in order to maintain high standards of practice, the teacher practitioners and mentors may become role models.

DRAWING PARALLELS AND FINDING RELATIONSHIPS

Perhaps one of the most significant elements here for teacher practitioners and mentors is in helping the learners to relate theory to practice, so that the natural separation between the two does not appear too wide to be bridged. It is, therefore, essential for teacher practitioners and mentors to try to keep abreast with developments in their field of practice, including the latest theoretical ideas, so that they can encourage their mentees and learners to be flexible in the light of new developments in order to ensure a high standard of practice.

REFLECTING FEELINGS

Practice in any caring profession involves an affective element, and teacher practitioners and mentors may have to help the students and junior colleagues cope with their emotions at two levels. In the first place, the practice itself may actually involve the learners in having to come to terms with their emotions in caring for their patients/clients. Teacher practitioners and mentors should be able to assist in this. For example, a student health visitor encountering a case of non-accidental injury to a child might feel angry towards the adults who inflicted it, a student nurse encountering death for the first time might feel distraught. In addition, students and new entrants to an occupation may also have emotional reactions to the learning processes that they themselves are undergoing, so that the teachers and mentors might have to help the students and junior staff come to terms with this aspect of their professional preparation. Sometimes current situations evoke memories of past traumatic experiences creating, or compounding, problematic situations. The more personal the relationship established between the two, the more this role is likely to become apparent. Teachers and mentors who are unable to cope with either their own or other people's emotions may be tempted to avoid any form of personal involvement with their students and mentees, so that these emotions do not surface in their presence. However, failure to help students and mentees at this level is a failure to perform one of the most important, but often neglected, aspects of professional preparation.

If teachers and mentors are prepared to acknowledge honestly their own emotions and reactions to stressful situations, especially when these have been previously suppressed, the students and mentees may then be willing to do likewise. The mere act of disclosure may create a valuable learning experience where the reasons why professionals react in a variety of ways to difficult encounters can be discussed. In addition, different ways of handling emotions can be considered together.

EXPRESSING AGREEMENT AND SUPPORT

It is significant that this is specified as a positive rather than a negative response to the learner. Since teacher practitioners and mentors are educators of adults they do have to help the learner know when she is correct and when she has made a mistake. However, one of the most stress-inducing responses that a learner can receive is to be told that she is wrong, rather than being helped to reach her own decision that she has made an error and that a specific aspect requires correction. Teachers and mentors should always express agreement when the students are correct and always offer support and guidance when they are in error. Praise and support need not always be verbal since a non-verbal response may be just as effective. Guidance may not always be in providing the correct answers but in helping the learners to think through the problem for themselves. This supportive environment is a factor of the teacher–learner relationship that was discussed above and which should constitute the basis for this teaching and developing process. Research demonstrates that praise and support produce greater advancement in the learning situation. Reproof, however, has the adverse effect. Carl Rogers (1969) actually concludes that anything but self appraisal may have harmful results.

FACILITATING CONTACTS

Increasing emphasis is being placed on self-directed learning, both in the context of initial training and in staff development thereafter. It is also being recognized that a great deal of expertise lies in practice and, therefore, experienced professional staff should be aware of the expertise of their colleagues and others in their fields of practice. Students and junior staff are not always aware of the richness of this expertise, nor do they always have the confidence to approach senior personnel, even if they are aware of their expertise. Both mentors and teacher practitioners are, therefore, resource persons in so much as they know the resources that their learners can use. They might be able to facilitate the type of contact that enables their learners or mentees to gain a great deal of new understanding. It is increasingly becoming an important role that senior staff can perform as workplaces get larger, more complex and diverse and more impersonal.

ADVICE AND GUIDANCE

The complexity of the workplace, the career opportunities that are available, the dilemmas that face junior staff are such that they do often need not so much a counsellor as a sounding board, one who can not only listen to their ideas and their problems but also provide some advice and guidance as a result. Where there is an excellent interpersonal relationship, teacher practitioners and mentors are likely to become advisers and guides. This is an important role for senior staff, although it is unwise for them to play a counselling role because this could interfere with the other aspects of professional practice. For young staff to know that there is a teacher practitioner or a mentor who has the time and commitment to listen to them is important in helping junior staff to try out new ideas and develop their own practice professionally. Additionally, in most of the caring professions in this time of economic stringency and tremendously heavy workloads, junior staff are being confronted with ethical dilemmas which they feel they need to discuss with someone who is more experienced but who is not necessarily in a management relationship to them. Mentors should be available for their mentees to enable such problems to be discussed openly without fear of any repercussions. It is also useful when junior staff reach crossroads in their own careers to know that there is a friend/mentor to whom they can turn for advice and guidance. For the mentoring relationship, when firmly established, can continue for many years.

Each of these roles has been mentioned here because it is an element in the interaction that will not occupy a significant place in the discussion hereafter. Yet each, in its own way, is vitally important to the teaching and learning process.

Conclusion

This chapter has begun to explore the teaching and learning interaction from the perspective of the teaching/mentoring role. It is maintained that an open honest dialogue between two human beings is at its heart: both bring themselves, their personalities and their experiences and both learn from each other. Both may share and both may be enriched. One of the privileges of the roles of teacher practitioner and mentor is that they can create a supportive environment in which fellow human beings can develop and acquire the knowledge, skills and attitudes appropriate to develop themselves in their chosen profession. Another is that the teacher practitioners and mentors may learn as much, or nearly as much, from the persons whom they teach, provided that an interactive relationship is established between the participants.

Having thus explored the teaching and learning interaction, it is now important that elements of student learning should be explored, so the next chapter focuses upon designing learning programmes for students. However, this aspect is clearly more relevant for teacher practitioners and mentors in structured course relationships than it is for the mentor who works with mentees beyond that period of initial preparation.

Designing a learning programme

3

This chapter explores:
- *The main elements of the curriculum*
- *Programme planning*
- *Needs and demands*
- *The notion of diagnosis*
- *Implementing and managing a learning programme.*

INTRODUCTION

This chapter focuses on the role of the teacher practitioner/preceptor/mentor in the more formal educational role of designing a learning programme for students, learners, etc. Consequently, it might be more applicable for teacher practitioners and preceptors than for those who perform an unstructured mentoring role.

Teacher practitioners and preceptors have two distinct functions in the design of a student's learning experiences:

- *as teachers* who perform a role within the broad framework of the curriculum that has been designated by the appropriate professional body and implemented in an approved teaching institution
- *as independent practitioners* responsible for designing a learning programme appropriate to the student's learning requirements within the practical experience component of professional preparation.

Consequently, teacher practitioners and preceptors need an understanding of the elements of curriculum theory and also some knowledge of the various approaches which can be employed in the design of learning programmes. Therefore, the first two sections of this chapter comprise a discussion of these aspects, since they give rise to the significant idea of 'need' and its relation to demand. Arising from this are the notions of learning needs, demand and diagnosis which are considered in turn. The final section elaborates some of the factors involved in implementing and managing a learning programme.

THE MAIN ELEMENTS OF THE CURRICULUM

The term 'curriculum' has a multitude of different meanings, so at the outset of this chapter it is necessary to establish a working definition. Many writers note this confusion of meanings; Kelly (1989 p10), for instance, points out that the term is employed to describe a variety of situations from the content of a particular subject or area of study to the total programme of an educational institution. The latter connotation is assumed here and Kerr's (1968 p16) widely accepted definition is adopted, so that the curriculum is taken to be 'all the learning which is planned and guided by the school, whether it is carried on in groups or individually, inside or outside of the school'. Since Kerr's work refers to initial education, as do many of the publications on curriculum, it is necessary to replace the term 'school' with that of 'educational institution'. Hence, the working definition of curriculum adopted here is: *all the learning which is planned and guided by the educational institution, whether it is carried on in groups or individually, inside or outside the institution.*

Significantly, there have been a number of writers more recently who have located their discussion on curriculum in the post-school framework since professional education has undergone considerable changes, and some reference is made to them below.

In addition to offering a variety of definitions, curriculum theorists categorize the various elements of the curriculum in different ways. Taba (1962 p422), for instance, proposed that one way of identifying these elements is to consider the major points at which decisions need to be taken in the process of curriculum development, and suggested that these are:

- aims and objectives
- content
- learning experiences
- evaluation.

Many curriculum theorists use these elements although 'learning experiences' is often replaced by 'teaching methods', in which both teaching and learning are emphasized, and 'evaluation' is sometimes recognized as including the assessment of learning outcomes, while in other schemes it is viewed as a separate entity from assessment.

The inter-relationship of these elements of the curriculum has been stressed for a number of years and, for example, Giles, McCutcheon and Zechiel (1942, cited in Taba 1962 p425) depict it as shown in Figure 3.1.

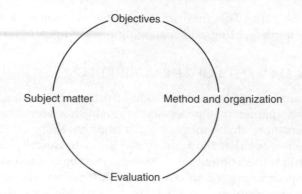

Figure 3.1   A model of the curriculum (following Giles *et al.*, 1942)

Taba points out that the design shown in Figure 3.1 describes the inter-relationship of these four elements but she stresses that for the curriculum developer it raises four questions:

1   What is to be done?
2   What subject matter is to be used?
3   What methods and organization are to be employed?
4   How are the results to be appraised?

While this model of curriculum is still employed, Nicholls and Nicholls (1978 p21) argue for 'a much wider and more comprehensive approach to diagnosis, an analysis of all the factors which make up the total situation followed by the use of knowledge and insights derived from this analysis in curriculum planning'. They stress the need for situation analysis to be a major stage in curriculum development and suggest the model shown in Figure 3.2.

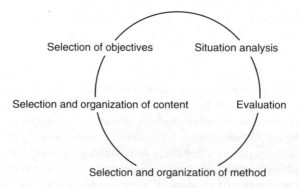
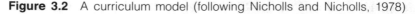

Figure 3.2   A curriculum model (following Nicholls and Nicholls, 1978)

However, this cyclical model (Figure 3.2) implies that everything occurs in sequence, whereas the selection and organization of content and method may occur concurrently during curriculum design.

One attractive approach to curriculum which has often been discussed, but not so frequently practised, is the spiral curriculum. Bruner (1977 p13) described this as a curriculum 'that turns back on itself at higher levels'. By this he meant that topics might be developed and re-developed at later times as the learners have acquired a greater capacity to understand the phenomenon. There is obviously a lot of sense in this approach since it allows for learner growth and reflection which also reflects a position argued by Kelly (1989 p69) that learning is developmental rather than linear. It is one which teacher practitioners, preceptors and mentors might use in a more informal approach to teaching and learning, building on the basic principles of practice and practical knowledge.

In recent years competency-based education has become the vogue in professional education, and in 1982 Blank produced a handbook in which he suggested there are 12 steps in preparing a competency-based training programme:

1 Identify and describe the occupation.
2 Identify the essential student pre-requisites.
3 Identify and verify job tasks.
4 Analyze job tasks and add necessary knowledge tasks.
5 Write terminal performance objectives.
6 Sequence tasks and terminal performance objectives.
7 Develop performance tests.
8 Develop written tests.
9 Develop draft learning guides.
10 Test and revise learning guides.
11 Develop a system to manage the learning.
12 Implement and evaluate training programme.

Clearly this is a very specific approach to training and for most people within the caring professions this is too skills-orientated. Additionally, it is very mechanistic and teacher-centred, so that it is not an approach that would be recommended here, although it does highlight certain specific points which might be incorporated into any curriculum preparation.

More recently, Bines (1992) suggested that professional education has had three different forms of curriculum: the pre-technocratic 'apprenticeship' model, the technocratic model and the post-technocratic model. The last of these is significant because it reflects the ethos of contemporary society, focusing specifically on knowledge for practice and competences. The teacher practitioner, whom she calls the practitioner educator, has a significant function in this formulation. Each of these models is examined under the following four headings:

- what is taught
- where it is taught
- who teaches it
- accountability.

It will be noted immediately that there is a different set of emphases in Bines' formulation than in the traditional approaches to curriculum and also in Blank's training approach. It might be asked, however, whether the original elements of curriculum no longer have a place in designing a curriculum. Naturally, this is not so, although a great deal of professional education has changed, so that it now necessary to be aware of the wider debate. These traditional categories and Bines' categories are now discussed sequentially in more detail.

AIMS AND OBJECTIVES

Aims are very general statements of goals and purposes, and they are usually expressed in abstract terms. They often provide a broad philosophical perspective for the curriculum and Davies (1976 p12) considers that an aim 'attempts to give both shape and direction to a set of more detailed intentions for the future'. He also suggests that an aim is 'an ideal, an aspiration, a direction in which to go'. Hence it may be seen that an aim is a general and long-term idea, whereas 'objectives' usually provide the actual direction over a more immediate time span. Reilly (1975 p8) points out that even though the goal may be defined, the route is not necessarily so clearly specified. However, objectives are more specific statements of the philosophical perspective and may be viewed as the means to achieving the long-term intention. Objectives may be expressed along two continua from general to specific, or from long-term to medium-term to short-term. Another early curriculum theorist, Wheeler (1967), refers to ultimate, mediate and proximate goals; with the ultimate goals being synonymous with the aims, the mediate ones relating to the specific development of a subject and the proximate relating to the direction of the individual lesson.

The pre-specification of aims and objectives, or whatever terminology is employed, is the result of educators attempting to provide direction for the development of the curriculum at every level. However, the desirability of providing such detailed direction is open to considerable question, especially since it proposes a teacher-centred learning model and this is not necessarily acceptable to educators of adults (see Robinson and Taylor, 1983). Learner-centred approaches have gained acceptance in a great deal of education for adults, although it must be recognized that some trainers find the approach epitomized by Blank as both rational and attractive. However, it is now recognized by many people that education is fundamentally about learning rather than teaching and that, ultimately, the teacher is not essential to the learning process. Hence, there has been a movement towards expressing objectives in learning rather than teaching terms, for example:

- educational objectives (Bloom, 1956)
- instructional objectives (Mager, 1975)
- behavioural objectives (Reilly, 1975)
- performance objectives (Davies, 1976)
- expressive objectives (Eisner in Popham *et al.*, 1969; Eisner, 1985).

It will be appreciated, therefore, that a number of different approaches might be recommended for producing specific objectives, since all of these stress learning outcomes. However, there are marked similarities between the first four of the aforementioned types, since all suggest that the objectives should specify the intended behaviour that the student should attain, the standards to be achieved and the conditions under which the behaviour will be manifest. These have become even more popular in recent years since there has been more emphasis on the practical outcomes of professional education in terms of competences. It will be suggested later in this section that some scholars consider that such precise prescription of desired behaviour is contrary to the ideals of adult education, unless these prescriptions have been negotiated between teacher and learner in advance, so that expressive objectives are much more in keeping with these ideals. Before discussing expressive objectives, it is necessary to explore some of the literature on objectives that relates to the other four types.

Educational and behavioural objectives may be specified in all three domains, i.e. cognitive (knowledge), affective (emotive, attitudinal) and psychomotor (skills), although they most frequently relate to the cognitive. Bloom *et al.* (1956) devised one of the most well known taxonomies of educational objectives in the cognitive domain, whilst Krathwohl *et al.* (1964) discussed one for the affective domain. More recently, Simpson (1966) and Harrow (1972) have been responsible for designing taxonomies in the psychomotor domain.

Bloom *et al.* suggest that there are six levels of knowledge:

1 *knowledge of specifics*, for example, terminology, facts
2 *comprehension*, for example, recipient is able to understand communication on specific topics
3 *application*, for example, ability to utilize specific knowledge to solve a problem

4 *analysis*, for example, ability to break down material into component parts and to detect inter-relationships
5 *synthesis*, for example, ability to draw together the parts to form a whole
6 *evaluation*, for example, ability to judge the value or purpose of ideas.

Bloom and his associates (1956 pp15–16) acknowledged that in producing the taxonomy in the cognitive domain they had been unable to produce a classification system that allowed for sharp distinctions in behaviour to be drawn and they recognized that complex behaviour is more than the sum of the more simple elements. That they placed so much emphasis on behaviour, even though they were writing in the cognitive domain, may now seem somewhat surprising, but this emphasis may have resulted in the popularity of the concept of behavioural objectives and the decline in emphasis being given to the term educational objectives. This taxonomy may be useful for the teacher practitioner to judge the appropriate levels of knowledge to which she should help the students aspire. The teacher practitioner utilizing the nursing, midwifery or health visiting process will appreciate the need to help students utilize knowledge at all levels if they are to acquire a professional approach to practice.

In this first study Bloom and associates concentrated upon the cognitive domain but, subsequently, Krathwohl *et al.* (1964) produced a second taxonomy in the affective domain and since teacher practitioners are involved in helping students acquire attitudes appropriate to working with people in stressful situations, this taxonomy is included here:

1 *reception*, for example, awareness, willingness to receive
2 *response*, for example, ability and willingness to respond and participate with others
3 *valuation*, for example, acceptance and commitment to values
4 *organization*, for example, organizing values into a system and recognition of the more important elements
5 *characterization*, for example, the unique set of values that make up individuality, a philosophy of life.

It will be noted by teacher practitioners that these values are really quite significant for professional practice since they encompass the way that professionals might be expected to relate both to their clients and to their peers. Krathwohl and his colleagues associate this taxonomy with the process of internalization and they (1964 p44) claim that 'as internalization progresses, the learner comes to attend to phenomena, to respond to them, to value and to conceptualize them'. They recognized that this process is akin to socialization, although not synonymous with it. The classification is useful, however, as a basis for understanding, and even assessing, one vital aspect of professional practice.

Bloom and his colleagues did not wish this separation into cognitive and affective domains to be regarded as indicating that they drew a fundamental separation between them in practice, rather they were seeking to provide a theoretical framework for educational objectives and a basis for assessment formulation. Teacher practitioners should not, therefore, overlook the basic unity of the two domains, but it will be recognized immediately that the setting of affective objectives in this manner may be interpreted as a form of indoctrination. But since professionalism itself has a moral basis, it might be argued that no profession should admit new recruits who have not had the opportunity to consider ethical issues underlying the practice of the profession and who embrace certain of them which they regard as basic to their own practice. Since social workers, nurses, midwives and health visitors are required to interact and care for patients and clients with impartiality, it could be maintained that it would be immoral to admit to practice those whose standards and values inhibit this. Thus teacher practitioners and preceptors should be aware of objectives in the affective domain and be prepared to utilize them appropriately in the teaching and learning interaction, since attitudes and values are included in some of the syllabi of their professions.

However, teacher practitioners are also teachers of skills and, while Bloom and his associates never devised a taxonomy of educational objectives in the psychomotor domain, at least two have been devised since the publication of their work. Harrow (1972) suggested that there are six levels of skill:

1 *reflex movements*, for example, to flex
2 *basic fundamental movements*, for example, to crawl
3 *perceptual abilities*, for example, to catch
4 *physical abilities*, for example, to move precisely
5 *skilled movements*, for example, to type
6 *non-discursive communication*, for example, utilization of skilled movements to express emotion.

While this taxonomy is a useful starting point in thinking about the psychomotor domain, Simpson's (1966) earlier taxonomy may be more useful to the teacher practitioner:

1 *perceptual ability*, for example, awareness through the senses
2 *readiness*, for example, knowing what to do and how to do it
3 *learning parts of a skill*, for example, by imitation, practice
4 *habitualization*, for example, internalization of a skill
5 *performing complex motor acts*, for example, automatic performance of co-ordinated skill
6 *adapting and originating*, for example, devising individual ways to skill performance according to individual perception.

It may thus be seen from Simpson's classification that one element in skills teaching is that of breaking the skill into its component parts, and then helping the learner acquire familiarity with each part. Learners should be allowed to practise skills at their own pace, as will be discussed in a later chapter. The final point that Simpson makes is that the highest level in skill performance is that of adaptation, so that it would be unwise for teacher practitioners or preceptors to expect that students will imitate them and then continue to perform the skill in precisely the way that it has been demonstrated. Indeed, adaptation is a vital element of reflective practice, since practitioners should always be monitoring their own practice and adapting it to the immediate needs and demands of the situation.

It is perhaps significant that in more recent work in higher education on improving the skills of graduates, many of these points appear in slightly different form. However, these are often listed as desired outcomes. One such formulation suggests that there are: core skills (personal skills – both about the self and in human interaction); self-management skills; other management skills; teamwork skills; skills in client interaction.

In addition, within the framework of National Vocational Qualifications, there are five levels of competence:

1   routine skills
2   a range of activities, not necessarily complicated, for which individual workers are required to take responsibility
3   a range of skills, many complicated, for which the workers have to take responsibility as they work alone and they may be required to guide the work of others
4   a wide range of technical or professional work for which the workers take responsibility for their own and others work
5   individuals organize, plan, design, check own and others' work.

Clearly this approach to education is becoming more prevalent, even though there are many people in education who consider this to be a rather limiting approach to the process of teaching and learning. Nevertheless, it is important that in planning curricula or educational programmes that teachers and mentors are aware of these new developments and relate their own work to them. Some further reference to these will be made in a later chapter.

Eisner (1985 pp29–37) objects to behavioural-type objectives for a variety of reasons, including the fact that the outcomes of learning are more complex than those specified in behavioural objectives models of the curriculum and that subject matters place their own constraints upon objectives. He concludes that methods of curriculum development make it an art form which requires creativity which the behaviourist approach fails to recognize. In earlier writings, he (in Popham *et al.*, 1969 p16) first made the point that the educational encounter between students and teachers is one in which it is impossible to specify outcomes. He (1969 p8) considers that the educational process 'enables individuals to behave intelligently through the exercise of judgments in situations that demand reflection, appraisal and choice among alternative courses of action'. Therefore, it is likely that the educational process will produce different learning outcomes for individual students. In such instances, behavioural objectives may be considered inappropriate and their morality needs to be questioned if they are forced upon learners; expressive objectives, therefore, might be more appropriate. These are in marked contrast to behavioural ones since they describe an educational encounter in which the student and teacher engage but do not specify its outcome. Eisner (in Popham *et al.*, 1969 p16) suggests that expressive objectives provide both teacher and student with the opportunity to explore issues that are significant to them but this approach is not prescriptive, since the individuality of the persons and the uniqueness of the experience should not result in homogeneity. Expressive objectives are not, therefore, intended as a common measure of learning outcomes, but a basis upon which lessons may be planned. They are, therefore, useful in the individualized learning situation where teacher practitioners and preceptors and the learner may share their experiences to their mutual enrichment, although it needs to be recognized that the responsibility for the teaching and learning transaction must remain with the former.

Another significant argument against the use of crude behavioural objectives in education and training lies in the fact that they tend to reflect a teacher-centred approach to teaching and learning, which specifies precisely what is to be learned and performed almost unthinkingly in the practice situation. If individual responsibility is to be encouraged in professional practice, then some form of responsibility needs to be given to the learner from the outset. Indeed, Reilly (1975 p9) considers goal setting to be a mutual responsibility since teachers and learners should have respect for each other and that engaging in such an exercise is both developmental and fulfilling.

While the morality of behavioural objectives has been questioned, there is a sense in which mutually-agreed behavioural objectives may have a place in skills training, but even these require negotiation. Hence in the education and training of professional practitioners, a combination of behavioural and expressive objectives may be appropriate, although the place of the latter should be more significant than that of the former.

CONTENT

In professional education the content of the curriculum is generally assumed to comprise the knowledge, skills and attitudes considered appropriate for practice, although some consideration might be given to the beliefs, ideologies and values of the caring services. In some situations the role for which the learner is being prepared has been fully analyzed and the different elements of the content identified, in rather the manner suggested by Blank's model of competencies discussed earlier in this chapter, and in these instances the curriculum may itself be based upon numerous specific objectives that will form a rationale for content selection. Alternatively, the curriculum developers may have relied solely upon aims, or general objectives, in producing an outline curriculum. In which case, the decision about what content to include, for example, appropriate knowledge, skills and attitudes, etc. and how to structure it, for example, multi-disciplinary or inter-disciplinary, thematic or modular, is the responsibility of the relevant educational establishment. When the selection of content has been made it is usually discussed internally by the relevant college or university bodies and then it is submitted to the statutory body, or validation body, or both, for external approval. The validation process is fully discussed in Chapter 7 so that no further reference will be made to it here. However, professional practice is frequently changing and teacher practitioners are in an ideal situation to ensure that new developments in their practice are reflected in new submissions for validation as part of the on-going process of curriculum development, so that it may be seen that they should be helping to ensure that the curriculum is always relevant to professional practice. This also indicates that often curriculum content follows professional practice rather than vice versa, and this reflects an important epistemological fact about practical knowledge – it must be practice-driven.

Since students differ in personality, ability, experiences and knowledge, their learning needs during their professional preparation differ, so that the actual content of any teaching and learning session should rarely be solely prescribed by either the document that was submitted for validation or the planners of the course. Hence, teacher practitioners and preceptors have some responsibility for the selection of content in the individual sessions that they teach. This is a responsibility that they may exercise in a variety of ways, including discussing with the students the areas that they consider should be covered. However they approach it, there are some teaching sessions in which they are responsible for structuring the content, so that it is most easily learned by the students and there are a number of points that they may find useful when doing this. The content should:

- be seen to be relevant to the student
- move from the known to the unknown
- develop from the simple to the complex
- develop from the concrete to the abstract
- develop from the particular to the general
- commence with the whole, sub-divide into the parts and then re-synthesize into the whole.

Thus it may be seen here that teacher practitioners will be able to relate theory to practice and practice to theory. In addition, it will be noted that this sequencing fits into the experiential learning theories that are discussed elsewhere in this text. Overall, it is suggested that this approach forms the basis of student-centred teaching that is relevant to the work of teacher practitioners and preceptors.

METHODS

Few curricula specify the precise teaching and learning strategies to be employed by the teaching staff responsible for their implementation, although some statutory bodies, for example, the English National Board, require information about the methods that are to be employed when the submission of the course is made. However, the type of information required is of a general, rather than specific, nature so that the teacher usually has freedom of choice in deciding what approaches to utilize. Naturally, the teacher's own philosophy and experience in teaching adults will influence the methods utilized but the learning objectives, the content and the situation will also exercise considerable influence upon the methods finally selected. Finally, the students themselves might express preferences that should be taken into consideration and discussed with them. Since teaching methods are discussed in a later chapter of this book no further reference to them will be made here.

EVALUATION

Evaluation means 'to place a value upon', so in the educational context it tends to be restricted to curriculum development, while assessment usually refers to the process of appraising students' abilities and achievements, and this latter term is discussed fully in Chapter 6.

Curriculum evaluation is a complex topic and space forbids detailed explanation of it here. However, it is widely regarded as the 'process of delineating, obtaining and providing information useful for making decisions and judgments' (Davis, 1980 p13) with a view to developing new curricula. It may be seen from Figure 3.2 that curriculum evaluation involves an examination of the appropriateness of the aims, objectives and content and of the effectiveness and appropriateness of the methods employed. The complexity of the subject becomes more apparent when it is recognized that there may be no agreed philosophy underlying all aspects of the course, little way of assessing the appropriateness of all the content to the work situation and only subjective means of measuring the effectiveness of the teaching methods employed or the learning experiences provided. Hence, there are no objective and universal standards of measurement and no accepted baselines from which the learning outcome can be appraised. Thus, the attractiveness of behavioural objectives might be seen, since they might be regarded as a baseline from which the effectiveness of the teaching and learning may be measured. But, as will be demonstrated in Chapter 4, behaviourism provides a false definition of learning, so that it is ultimately a weak support in the process of evaluation. Over the past two decades, the concept of illuminative evaluation has become more popular with curriculum theorists: this approach enables evaluators to make their own subjective assessment of the processes which they have observed and which allows the recipients of the evaluation to make their own decision about the curriculum (see Hamilton 1976 p39).

More recently, naturalistic approaches to curriculum evaluation have been utilized (see Guba and Lincoln, 1981) which have recognized that it is problematic to appear to be dealing with objective facts rather than more personal perspectives in this exercise.

Frequently, tutors seek an evaluation from their students of the course in which they have participated and this is often conducted at the end of the course by means of a questionnaire. While there is a certain value in this approach, although this is rarely discussed but rather assumed, it must be remembered that this is an immediate evaluation of a process which may also have long-term effects, so that it may be more relevant to evaluate the course twice. Initially, immediately after it has been completed and then again a few months later when the new recruits are fully established in practice. This is even more important when the course being evaluated is in-service, continuing professional education, since one of the main reasons for such courses is to assist the practitioners to learn new knowledge and skills, etc. (see Robinson and Robinson, 1989). This is the beginning of impact evaluation – naturally, employers and senior colleagues can also contribute to this process. At the same time it must be recognized that students continue to learn once they enter practice and impact evaluation tends to play down the process of continuing learning.

Each of the elements of the traditional curriculum approach have now been examined briefly in order to highlight the theory underlying the course in which the teacher practitioners are involved. However, it is also important to look at the four dimensions that Bines cited (see page 38) in order to broaden the perspectives on curriculum design:

WHAT IS TAUGHT

Bines specifies that this must be knowledge for practice with an emphasis on competences. The concept of practical knowledge has already been explored and this is in accord with Bines' approach. Clearly there has been a considerable emphasis on competences in recent years and, while this is perfectly correct in as far as it goes, it must be remembered that the nature of practice is more than the sum of its parts, and the nature of education is far broader than competency-based.

Bines also specifies the need to develop systematic reflection and while the need to understand reflective learning is recognized here, it might be wiser to broaden this idea and recognize that there is a genuine need to help practitioners and recruits 'learn how to learn' (Smith, 1982).

Finally, Bines highlights the need to learn some research skills and it is wise to recognize that every practitioner should be a researcher through the process of reflective practice, and systematic reflection should lead to systematic research in practice. As long ago as 1975, Stenhouse made a plea for all teachers to be researchers and the ideas of action research are conducive to both teachers and professional practioners being researchers of their own practice.

WHERE IT IS TAUGHT

Bines points out that the practice situation is the key place to develop competence, and this is so. However, it must be pointed out here that clinical practice is not a matter of applying theory to practice, but it is a matter of learning how to practise as a result of having gained some previous knowledge.

WHO TEACHES IT

Bines recognizes that teacher practitioners and perceptors play a significant role here in promoting reflective practice, in relationship with professional tutors. Clearly this is an important statement, but when she also claims that subject specialists should be eliminated she is probably overstating her position, especially when she adds that there might actually be a negotiated role for them based upon their professional credibility.

ACCOUNTABILITY

This is a significantly new concept in curriculum design in as much as it changes the emphasis from evaluation – now course teams are accountable, usually to a partnership of employing agency and higher education institutions. At the same time, there is another sense in which they should be accountable to themselves and their students.

Since they are teachers, as well as practitioners, and they are increasingly expected to play a role within the educational institution and even be involved in curriculum design, it is also essential that both teacher practitioners and preceptors understand the way in which learning programmes are designed and so the next part of this chapter examines programme planning.

PROGRAMME PLANNING

The distinction between curriculum and programme has been explored elsewhere (Jarvis, 1995a: 189–92) and so this will not be discussed fully here. Suffice it to note that a programme consists of a number of courses, usually called modules, which form a menu from which learners can choose to study the ones which they need, or want, to study. As education is becoming a marketable commodity, so the modular structure is becoming increasingly functional. The market also needs to be able to award credit for prior learning – both accrediting prior learning (APL) and accrediting prior experiential learning (APEL) – and transferring credit. In addition, it also has to respond to the more precise needs of the purchasers, so that the more traditional curriculum approaches to educational provision are threatened. Since initial professional preparation tends to prescibe a great deal of what is taught, the modular structure can be less flexible. In professional continuing education, however, it can function in a more flexible manner. Clearly, such approaches are functional but whether they are always epistemologically justifiable is a more open question.

Teacher practitioners and preceptors might well be involved in preparing individual modules, but the focus of this section is upon the process of preparing the whole menu, or programme. Blank's (1982) model approximates to some of the American models of programme planning and these have relevance for teachers concerned with either type of provision, so that some aspects of these are now considered.

From a large volume of literature published on the topic in the United States, there are according to Long (1983 p158) four most frequently cited stages in designing a learning experience:

1 determine the training needs
2 design the programme

3   provide the instruction
4   evaluate the programme.

It may be seen that these four points have considerable similarity with the different aspects of the curriculum discussed above, especially if the teacher's objectives are to endeavour to respond to the student's needs. Two other well known approaches are mentioned here: Houle's (1972) model has nine stages and Boone's (1985) approach has five. Houle specified the following stages:

1   identification of a possible educational programme
2   decision to proceed
3   identification of objectives
4   refining objectives
5   designing a format
6   contextualizing a format
7   putting the plan into operation
8   measuring the results
9   evaluating the results.

Houle recognized that in designing the format it is necessary to consider: resources; leaders; methods; sequence; social reinforcement; individualization; roles and relationships; criteria for evaluation; clarity of design. In addition, he suggested that when contextualizing the format, planners had to consider: guidance or counselling; lifestyle; finance; interpretation.
   In contrast to this, Boone's five stages are:

1   understanding the organization within which the programme is to be conducted
2   linking the organization to its publics
3   designing the programme
4   implementing the programme
5   evaluating the programme and accounting for it.

However, it will be noted that all of these approaches assume that the educational activity is teacher-initiated and designed. This is less true of the model constructed by Knowles (1980 pp223–47), whose learner-centred model is:

1   set a climate for learning
2   establish a structure for mutual planning
3   diagnose needs for learning
4   formulate directions (objectives) for learning
5   design a pattern of learning experiences
6   manage the execution of the learning experiences
7   evaluate the results
8   rediagnose the learning needs.

Knowles' approach relates more closely to the one advocated here than to the teacher-initiated ones mentioned above. It will be seen immediately that Knowles' first step is very similar to that discussed in the previous chapter, when the importance of establishing a good relationship with the student was highlighted. However, it is the second point that requires emphasis here: while the teacher practitioners and preceptors may know in their own mind what they think the students ought to learn, they must also recognize that as adults (and possibly as experienced nurses, health visitors, midwives and social workers) the students might also know what they want, or think they need, to learn. Therefore, it is maintained that the design of the students' learning experience should emerge after a period of mutual planning. This does not mean that the teacher practitioners and preceptors merely provide what the students wish to learn, but that in a negotiated situation both participants plan the learning experience. Hence, the diagnosis of learning needs and the formulation of learning objectives may emerge from a mutual planning exercise. This spirit of mutuality should, provided that the interpersonal relationship initially established is maintained, prevail through all the stages of the learning experiences that teacher practitioners and preceptors facilitate for the students.

Long (1983 p164) claims that no research known to him has actually tested Knowles' model, but Jarvis and Gibson (1980 pp71–4) discovered that practical work teachers and student district nurses, who did not undertake a period of mutual planning, often had completely different aims for the same period of professional practical experience. Hence, this time of professional practice had not resulted in such a rich teaching and learning experience as it might have done had there been some joint planning. Knowles does employ two other concepts in his model of designing learning experiences that require further elucidation: needs and diagnosis. However, as education has become a marketable commodity and the provision of continuing education, especially, has changed quite dramatically in recent years, it is necessary to consider needs in the wider context of demands. Hence, the next two parts of this chapter considers needs, demands and diagnosis. The final section examines the process of implementing and managing a learning programme.

NEEDS AND DEMANDS

It will have become apparent from the discussion above that the learner and the teacher practitioner may perceive the student's needs in differing ways. This indicates one of the major problems of the concept of 'need' in education; it is used in a variety of ways by different participants in the educational process and even by different scholars. Many teacher practitioners will be familiar with Maslow's hierarchy of needs (Figure 3.3).

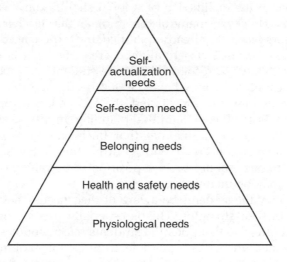

Figure 3.3 Maslow's Hierarchy of Needs (Maslow, 1968)

While Maslow's model has proved a helpful starting point for many discussions about the subject, it certainly does not exhaust the debate (see Jarvis 1995a pp11–15). Additionally, Hirst and Peters (1970 p33) suggest that there are needs of a diagnostic, biological, psychological basic and functional type, whilst Bradshaw (1972) considers that there are normative, felt, expressed and comparative needs. Hence, it may be seen that the concept itself is complex and confused.

Lawson (1975 p37) tried to clarify the debate when he suggested that 'a deficiency [that] can be remedied by the help of some educational process' may be regarded as an educational need. This is a useful definition in many ways because it specifies a type of need, but 'education' is a much more difficult term to define. Even more problematic in this definition is the implication that educational processes are always designed to remedy a deficiency rather than to respond to wants or interests. More recently, it has been suggested by some writers (for example Illich, 1977; Armstrong, 1982) that the concept is ideological. The reason for this view is that learning needs are frequently defined from above, i.e. it is the teacher or professional body which defines the need, rather than from below, i.e. the learner. This accusation certainly appears to have some validity since it is usually assumed that the professional is the person to diagnose and the client/patient is a passive recipient of the diagnosis.

This also appears to be true for traditional education, and it might be argued that in the case of children there is every justification for this approach. A similar perspective might be presented in professional education, since the qualified professional should know what the new recruit needs. However, many of the students that teacher practitioners and preceptors teach are already qualified and experienced professional practitioners, albeit in a closely aligned area. Hence, it is necessary for teacher practitioners to recognize that the students may be very aware of deficiencies that they may have, i.e. felt needs, and that they may be prepared to express them provided that the relationship established between them is conducive to mutual planning. In these instances, needs are not ideological in the manner that Illich and Armstrong suggest, since they are not concerned with control. But at the same time the teacher practitioner should be in a position to perceive needs of which the student may be unaware.

Not only may the students be aware of their needs, they may also be well aware of their strengths. This is especially true in continuing professional education so that potential students select modules according to their own wants, where this is possible, from the menu of modules in the new forms of course provision. This, therefore, raises the question of demand – an economic concept that is frequently coupled with the supply. Educational organizations are now often expected to offer modules on the educational market and see whether there is suffcent demand to justify running it. This approach to education has caused a great deal of heart searching among some educators in recent years, although this has always been an accepted approach in liberal adult education classes. One of the major problems with this approach, however, is when those who operate according to the market confuse their activities with the language of 'needs' since this diverts people from the actual nature of the activity. Nevertheless, even in the market-type situation, teachers and preceptors can still diagnose the learning needs of those who enrol in their classes.

THE NOTION OF DIAGNOSIS

Knowles refers to this as diagnosing learning needs, whereas other writers, such as Rowntree (1977), discuss a similar concept under the title of formative assessment. Rowntree (1977 pp121–2) states that formative assessment occurs when the teacher intends to use 'the knowledge he [sic] gains about the student . . . diagnostically [in helping] the student grow'. Hence, diagnostic appraisal is a teaching tool. It has been suggested elsewhere (Jarvis, 1979) that if teacher practitioners are to use the limited time available to them to the best possible advantage, they should undertake a diagnostic appraisal of the student's work very early in the period of time allocated to professional practice.

This approach to diagnosis of needs requires the teacher practitioner and the student to identify jointly those areas in which the student is already proficient and those in which further assistance will be required. Obviously there may be instances where teacher practitioners and preceptors wish to assess the student's level of knowledge, skills and attitudes in order to decide whether they think that the student is proficient, since they may have different standards to those of the students. The teacher practitioners would then be in a position to discuss with the learners what they consider to be the students' learning needs, and they can then negotiate together the areas in which further teaching and learning should occur. Thus it may be seen that, since adult learners bring certain skills and experiences to the individualized teaching and learning situation, the programme should be prepared to respond to the teaching and learning needs jointly agreed upon by both teacher practitioner and student. Diagnosis should be undertaken during the early stage of the teaching and learning programme, and it should then become an on-going process. Whilst teacher practitioners should regard themselves as diagnosticians, they should not automatically or autocratically prescribe the educational remedy for the diagnosis. They should, however, be prepared to discuss their diagnosis with the learners, who might also have felt needs in these areas or even disagree with the diagnosis and wish to discuss it further. Therefore, the teaching and learning programme may be something that is both mutually agreed but flexible enough to allow for development or modification, depending upon the learning needs of the students as perceived by both the learners and the teacher practitioners or preceptors. The idea of mutual planning is also known as a negotiated curriculum, but the difference between it and many other negotiated curricula is that in this instance the negotiation should be an on-going process throughout the whole of the teaching and learning period and not something that occurs once only at the outset of the programme.

Whilst 'needs' are a useful basis for programme planning, teacher practitioners and students must ensure that all aspects of the content of the curriculum are covered during the professional practical experience, and that they are dealt with in the appropriate depth and breadth in relation to those needs. In addition, it must be recognized that many of them can be met by the teacher assuming the role of facilitator and the students becoming more self-directed.

IMPLEMENTING AND MANAGING A LEARNING PROGRAMME

From what has been discussed so far in this chapter, it may be seen that, in individualized teaching and learning in the education of adults, it is advocated that the planning process should be a mutual undertaking between the teacher practitioners and preceptors and the learners. However, it is recognized that the approach suggested here is an ideal one and that it is not always possible to implement. On occasions, teacher practitioners may have had little time to discuss everything with the learners. On other occasions, they may endeavour to act independently of the learners for a variety of reasons, although it is emphasized here that this should be the exception rather than the rule. Nevertheless, even in this situation of mutuality, it must be recognized that it is still the teacher practitioners' responsibility to provide the teaching or facilitation through which the learning may occur. Davies (1971 pp22–30) equates the teacher to a manager and he coined the term teacher manager and, while the term is not totally acceptable here, since it implies a form of authority other than that of the professional, it is realistic to recognize that there are sufficient similarities between the ideas of teacher and manager to allow for comparison. Davies, for instance, points out that there are four management functions that are appropriate to teaching: planning, organizing, leading and controlling. Thus far it has been advocated that the planning should be a mutual exercise, whenever possible, between two human beings each seeking to maximize the potential of the interaction. Clearly, when teacher practitioners have resources at their disposal they should organize them in order to achieve the objectives that have been agreed. The teaching and learning strategies that they choose and the teaching and learning aids that they prepare may all be regarded as part of the process. Davies suggests that teaching may be related to motivating, encouraging and inspiring learners, and in this sense, it relates both to the quality of the interpersonal relationship established and to the professionalism of the teacher practitioners and preceptors which may inspire the learners to seek to achieve similar standards. Finally, Davies equates controlling to monitoring the learning and adjusting the process if it is not as efficient as it might be. In this manner, teacher practitioners and preceptors may be regarded as managing the learning experience, but perhaps Knowles' (1980 p239) description of the teacher is a little more appropriate to the role of the teacher practitioner in implementing and managing the learning experience:

> The role of the teacher in this phase . . . is to serve both as a strong procedural technician . . . suggesting the most effective ways the students can help in executing the decisions (how to implement strategies of learning into effective learning situations) – and as a resource person or coach, who provides substantial information regarding the subject matter of the unit, possible techniques and available materials where needed. The leader can also perform a

useful 'threading' function, providing the connective tissue or transitional commentary from one unit to the next.

While Knowles acknowledges that the teacher does manage the teaching and learning interaction, he emphasizes the role of the learner far more than does Davies and is, therefore, much more in accord with the approach to teaching and learning that is advocated here. Even so, it cannot be emphasized enough that however successful the interpersonal relations between the teacher practitioners and learners, the former remains responsible for achieving effectively the overall aim of this element in the professional preparation of each student.

Conclusion

This chapter has begun to explore some of the main issues that indicate the design of a learning programme and perhaps can be summarized by expanding Knowles' 'andragogical model' of the teacher whose role is to:

- set the climate by establishing good interpersonal relations from the outset
- establish a structure of mutual planning, so that:
  - the overall aim of the professional practice is recognized
  - procedures for discussion about progress are decided
  - procedures for planning the professional experience are agreed upon
- diagnose learning needs by:
  - listening to the learner express the needs that she recognizes
  - assessing her practice and diagnosing her strengths and weaknesses
  - agreeing together on the areas of strength and need
- formulate objectives for learning by mutual planning
- design a pattern of learning experiences by:
  - selecting appropriate teaching methods/learning experiences
  - effective utilization of all resources, including colleagues and their caseloads, as appropriate
- manage the learning experiences by:
  - implementing the plan
  - monitoring the process
- evaluate the results by:
  - discussion with the learner about both the process and her own assessment of what she has gained
  - observation of the product, where appropriate

- rediagnose the learning needs by:
    - listening to the learner express the needs that she recognizes
    - assessing her practice and diagnosing the strengths and needs
    - agreeing together on the areas of strength and need.

Thereafter the process should begin again, so that teacher practitioners and preceptors are continually redesigning the plans for the programme to ensure that by the end of the period of professional practice its overall aim will have been achieved.

Adult learning 4

This chapter explores:
- *Some theories of learning*
- *The learning cycle*
- *Adult learning and andragogy*
- *Cognitive learning styles*
- *Learning in the affective domain*
- *Learning skills*
- *Learning how to learn.*

INTRODUCTION

Learning may be defined as 'the transformation of experience into knowledge, skills, attitudes, emotions, values, beliefs, senses, etc.' This is an experiential definition upon which much of this book is based (see Jarvis, 1987; 1992; 1995a for more detail). At the same time, it is important to note that all learning begins with experience and that an experiential definition illustrates the significance of teacher practitioners, mentors and preceptors since they are frequently the providers or facilitators of the professional experiences from which learning in the workplace begins.

It may be noted immediately that this definition differs from many others which emphasize a change in behaviour, for example, learning is 'a relatively permanent change in behaviour that occurs as a result of practice' (Hilgard and Atkinson 1967 p270). This latter definition, frequently cited, highlights only behaviour modification whereas the former is less restrictive embracing, among others, the cognitive, affective and psychomotor domains. The importance of the emotions has been highlighted by Boud *et al.* (1985), and Mezirow (1991) has emphasized the ways that personal meaning is transformed through learning. Learning is, therefore, a broader phenomenon than that implied by the behavioural or cognitive definitions.

That adults have ability to learn has never been denied although it has been assumed frequently that learning is mainly undertaken in childhood and that the ability to learn, and also intelligence, decline as the adult ages. However, as early as 1928 Thorndike *et al.* could conclude that the research until then would lead them to estimate that 'adult ability to learn [is] very close to that of the late teens' (Thorndike *et al.*, 1928 p31). Research in more recent years, however, has suggested that the age limit on learning performance may not occur before 75 years (Cross, 1981 p154), so the adage that 'old dogs cannot learn new tricks' is a myth that needs to be laid to rest. Indeed, the idea of the European Year of Lifelong Learning, in 1996, emphasizes the fact that learning is both a lifelong and a lifewide phenomenon. Even more recently the Delors Report (1996) has placed considerable emphases on lifelong learning in the context of both work and general living. The growth in Universities of the Third Age illustrate that the desire to learn, even the most academic subjects, is not necessarily quelled with age.

However, it has also been suggested that the methods by which adults learn change, so that it is incumbent for teacher practitioners, mentors and preceptors to be aware of recent research findings in this area to ensure that they become more effective teachers, since they will work with learners from across a wide age range.

Learning, then, is a lifelong process, but it is useful to know some of the theoretical perspectives about it, so the first section of this chapter contains a very brief summary of some of the main theories. The weaknesses of some of these approaches are highlighted in an examination of an experiential learning cycle. Thereafter, the concepts of adulthood and adult development are discussed and it is recognized that adults bring different characteristics to bear upon learning.

Learning in the cognitive, affective and psychomotor domains is considered thereafter, and the chapter concludes with a summary of those elements discussed herein which are known to enhance or inhibit adult learning.

SOME THEORIES OF LEARNING

A number of theories of learning have been propounded over the years. All of them have value but one of the major weaknesses that many of them have is that the research upon which they are based has been conducted with animals rather than developed with adults. Consequently they are not completely satisfactory as explanations of adult learning. Three broad areas are mentioned here: connectionism, conditioning and gestalt theory. Experiential learning will be discussed thereafter.

CONNECTIONISM

Connectionism is frequently referred to as 'stimulus-response' learning and was developed by Thorndike (1898; 1911; 1913), whose research was conducted with cats, dogs and chickens. His research led him to three laws of learning, which he believed applied equally well to humans as to animals. These are the laws of:

- *readiness* – the circumstances under which the learner is satisfied, annoyed, etc.
- *effect* – the bond between stimulus and response is strengthened or weakened because of the level of emotive satisfaction that accompanies the action
- *exercise* – repetition of meaningful actions results in substantial learning readiness; if the organism is ready for the connection then the result is pleasurable and learning is increased but, if not, then the opposite result occurs.

Thorndike was later to revise his work on the law of effect and the law of exercise was discarded. Nevertheless, his work was to have a profound effect on behaviourist theories of learning and there are elements of learning in these laws that are important for teacher practitioners to consider, for example:

- The greater the pleasure obtained from the learning experience, the more learning that will occur.
- The more meaningful the act to the student, the greater will be the resultant learning.
- Practice makes perfect, provided that the action is seen to be meaningful.

Pleasure and relevance are important elements in learning and in the teaching and learning interaction both should occur if learning is to be enhanced.

CONDITIONING

Both forms of conditioning are well known – *classical* and *operant*. Classical conditioning is associated with the work of Pavlov, who demonstrated that behaviour could be initiated by a stimulus. He showed that a dog could be made to salivate to the sound of a bell, provided that on a number of previous occasions the sound had been presented simultaneously with food. However, salivation will only occur for as long as the dog associates the sound with the food. Hence, it may be seen that in classical conditioning the process commences with an already well established response to a stimulus and the response is then associated with a different stimulus. This process occurs in therapy, when the patient may be conditioned by the therapist to acquire approved behavioural responses to specific stimuli, but it does appear to be a matter of reflex rather than cognitive learning.

Perhaps Skinner's operant conditioning, equally well known, has more applicability to education. He experimented with both rats and pigeons and demonstrated that, by rewarding acceptable behaviour, both could be taught to perform the type of behaviour that the experimenter wished them to learn; even relatively complicated behaviour could be taught by rewarding correct performance at each stage in its development. From his experiments, Skinner concluded that:

- learning could be maximized by positive reinforcement
- each stage in a complicated process needs to be restricted and grow out of previously learned behaviour
- reward should immediately be given after correctly learned behaviour
- the learner should be provided with the opportunity to discover behaviour that is not rewarded.

In this above formulation, it is possible to see how skills might be taught by breaking the procedure into a number of manageable sections, and helping the students to learn each stage in the sequence by individually rewarding each correct performance. Reward should be forthcoming in the shape of praise, etc., which is a substitute for the sweets and stars sometimes given to children for good behaviour or achievement. In the same way as skills can be taught by this approach, so cognitive and affective response can be learned. However, the extent to which conditioning is an educational process is open to debate. Nevertheless, it is a method of maximizing learning, and positive reinforcement is a weapon in every teacher's armoury. Additionally, it is a very important element in individualized teaching and learning in order to enhance the personal relationship that has been established between the teacher practitioners, mentors and preceptors and the learners. Additionally, it may be seen that operant conditioning may occur both in programmed learning and therapy.

GESTALT THEORY

Gestalt psychologists have tended to use apes or gorillas in their research and they have shown that these animals have been able to grasp patterns of actions when seeking to solve a problem. From these experiments it has been possible to suggest that the solutions:

- appear to occur by inspiration or insight as a result of perceived relationships within a given situation
- are permanent to that situation.

Clearly some people appear to respond to learning situations best when they have a holistic perspective, so that this approach to learning might well reflect one learning style. Hence, it may be seen that it may be beneficial for adult students to be presented with a meaningful whole in the first instance rather than isolated elements.

It would be possible to extend this discussion considerably but this is not within the scope of this small text, although further references are given in the recommended reading list at the end of this book.

THE LEARNING CYCLE

From the above section, it may be concluded that the more developed the species of animal, the greater the theory of learning appears to rely upon the active involvement of the learners. Hence, it is suggested here that human learning frequently involves something other than a reflex action acquired in response to a stimulus, but that it demands a process of active thought by the learner. This active involvement may occur in the form of reflection upon an experience, a problem or a situation and this may be presented in the form of a *learning cycle*. Much of the work on learning cycles has been developed by exponents of experiential learning, although it is maintained here that the learning process is similar, irrespective of the dimension in which the experience occurs. Additionally, it is important to recognize that there is an inter-relationship between the cognitive, affective and psychomotor dimensions and that changes in one of them may, but need not necessarily, result in changes in the other two.

One learning cycle frequently cited is that devised by Kolb and Fry (1975 pp33–7) (see Figure 4.1). It is presented here in its simple, initial formulation and then developed. Kolb maintained that the

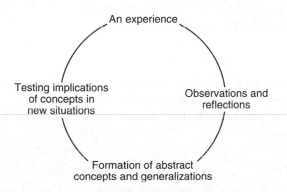

Figure 4.1   An experiential learning cycle (following Kolb and Fry, 1975)

learning process can begin anywhere on the cycle and then go through the subsequent stages.

Kolb's cycle has been extremely influential in many ways in recent years but subsequent research on it has demonstrated that it is over-simplified and learning from experience is actually not a single process but a number of diverse processes. Jarvis (1987) conducted research with adult learners, employing Kolb's cycle as part of the experimental process and he discovered the much more complex set of processes shown in Figure 4.2.

It may be seen from Figure 4.2, which is not as comprehensive as it might be, that there are a number of basic routes through, which indicate a number of different forms of learning response to experience: non-learning, non-reflective learning and reflective learning. Basically, there are at least nine different responses to experience, which have been typified as different forms of learning (see Table 4.1).

Table 4.1   A typology of learning

Category of response to experience	Type of learning/ non-learning	Route through diagram
Non-learning	Presumption	1–4
	Non-consideration	1–4
	Rejection	1–3, 7, 4 or 9
Non-reflective learning	Preconscious learning	1–3, 6, 4
	Skills learning	1–3, 5, 8, 6, 4 or 9
	Memorization	1–3, 6, 4 or 9
Reflective learning	Contemplation	1–3, 7, 8, 6, 9
	Reflective skills learning	1–3, 5, 7, 5, 8, etc., 6, 9
	Experimental learning	1–3, 7, 5, 7, 8, etc., 6, 9

It is now necessary to examine these different forms of learning and non-learning in order to relate them more closely to the work of teacher practitioners, preceptors and mentors.

NON-LEARNING

It is very clear that people do not always learn from their experiences and so the first group of responses are non-learning ones: presumption, non-consideration and rejection. Each of these three sub-types are now described briefly.

Presumption

Presumption is the rather typical response to everyday experience. Schutz and Luckmann (1974 p7) describe it thus:

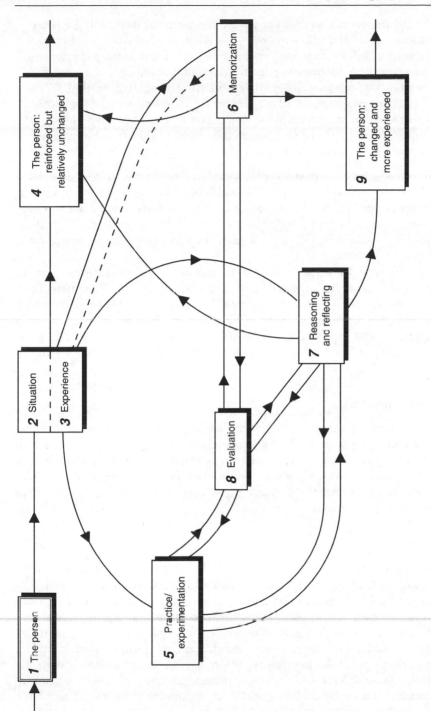

Figure 4.2 A model of the learning processes (Jarvis, 1987)

I trust the world as it is known by me up until now will continue further and that consequently the stock of knowledge obtained from my fellow-men [*sic*] and formed from my own experiences will continue to preserve its fundamental validity ... From this assumption follows the further and fundamental one; that I can repeat my past successful acts. So long as the structure of the world can be taken as constant; so long as my previous experience is valid, my ability to operate upon the world in this and that manner remains in principle preserved.

While this appears almost thoughtless and mechanical, it is suggested here that this is the basis of all social living. It would be quite intolerable for people to have to consider every word and every act in every social situation before they undertook it. Hence, a great deal of life is lived on the basis of previous learned experiences and presumption is a typical response.

In addition, to achieve this state has been the traditional aim of training, since it has always been regarded as more efficient to have workers who could perform their skills without having to think about them. Such an approach in nursing or social work is, however, extremely dangerous and is most likely to produce bad practice, so that basic approaches to training are less frequently applicable to nursing or social work!

Non-consideration

For a variety of reasons people do not respond to a potential learning experience; maybe because they are too busy to think about it, and it is very easy to think of work situations where this occurs. Thus it may be seen that non-consideration is another non-learning response that occurs quite commonly in both work and everyday life to potential learning experiences.

Rejection

Some people have an experience, think about it but reject the possibility of learning that could have accompanied the experience. For instance, think of an elderly person experiencing the complexity of modern society and exclaiming, 'I don't know what this world is coming to these days!' Here is a possible learning experience, an experience of the complex modern world, but instead of probing it and seeking to understand it, the person rejects the possibility. While the illustration here is with the elderly, it could have been with the not so elderly; with bigots or fundamentalists who look at the world and exclaim that they will not have any opinion or attitude changed by it, etc.

But there is another way of looking at this: the experienced practitioners who know that their way works and who have confidence in their own skills are likely to reject some new theories to which they are introduced, until it can be demonstrated to them that the new approach is better. Sometimes practitioners are regarded as conservative by teachers and theorists just because they do not jump at the chance of introducing new approaches – but the practitioners' practical knowledge and skills might have been learned from reflecting on experience and experimenting in a rigorous manner, so that there might be a tendency to reject something new unless it can be demonstrated to be better. In this case, the rejection might be perfectly justified because of the professionalism of the practitioners.

NON-REFLECTIVE LEARNING

These forms of learning are those which are most frequently socially defined as learning. For the sake of convenience the three that have been isolated in the research underlying this section of the chapter (Jarvis, 1987) are: preconscious, skills learning and memorization. The factor, above all else, that enables them to be placed within one stratum together is that they do not involve reflectivity.

Preconscious learning

There is little research into this form of learning. It occurs to everybody as a result of their having experiences in the course of their daily life about which they do not really think and about which they are not even particularly conscious. They occur at the periphery of the vision, at the edge of consciousness, etc. Ruth Beard (1976 pp93–5) calls this incidental learning and she suggests that people develop such phenomena as schemas of perception as a result of these experiences. Other scholars who have been interested in this approach include Mannings (1986), who researched incidental learning in an adult education institution, and Reischmann (1986), who presented a paper at American Association of Adult and Continuing Education in which he talked about learning *en passant*. Now this research project was not itself aimed at analyzing this type of learning, although a number of the respondents mentioned this possibility during the research itself. It is similar in approach to the next two forms of learning.

Skills learning

This is traditionally restricted to such forms of learning as training for a manual occupation or the acquisition of a high level of physical fitness through training or drill. However, some learning in preparation for a manual occupation is certainly not non-reflective, so this has to be restricted to the learning of simple, short procedures that somebody on an assembly line might be taught. These skills are often acquired through imitation and role modelling.

Memorization

This is the most commonly known form of learning. Children learn their mathematical tables, their language vocabularies, etc. in this way. Adults, when they return to further or higher education, sometimes feel that this is the type of learning that is expected of them and so they try to memorize what such and such a scholar has written, etc. so that they can reproduce it in an examination. Hence, the authority speaks and every word of wisdom has to be learned – memorized. This approach has to be given less prominence by teacher practitioners and preceptors.

The significance of these approaches to learning in the wider social context become very clear. As long as these approaches to learning are practised, then learning is nothing more than a process of reproduction. The profession and its practices remain unquestioned and, consequently, unaltered. New recruits learn and as a result they fit easily into the larger organization or the wider society – they learn their place, as it were. Once again, this may be examined from the position of the individual and the wider society. Individuals who learn this way do learn to fit into the organization or society, through a process of socialization. In a rather simple recent study, from an anthroplogical perspective, Lave and Wenger (1991) wrongly viewed this process as a new radical approach to learning theory. However, McKenzie (1990) undertook a much more thorough and systematic analysis of this process with district nurses.

REFLECTIVE LEARNING

Thus far it has been shown that learning tends to be reproductive, simply because that is the way that it is frequently defined socially. It was suggested that non-reflective learning could not do other than reproduce the social structures of society, but this is not true of reflective learning. These forms of learning involve the process of reflection, and thinkers such as Freire (1972a; 1972b *inter alia*), Mezirow (1977; 1981), Argyris (1982 *inter alia*), Schon (1983 *inter alia*), Kolb (1984) and Boud *et al.* (1985) have all examined the process of reflection. Because of Freire's work it might be assumed that all reflective learning has to be revolutionary, but this must not be assumed to be the case. Reflective learning is not automatically innovative. But before this is discussed it is necessary to examine the three types of reflective learning that were isolated during the research which was mentioned previously (Jarvis, 1987): contemplation, reflective skills learning and experimental learning.

Contemplation

This is a form of learning that behaviourist definitions of the phenomenon make no allowance for and yet, in many ways, this might be viewed as a very intellectual approach to learning because it involves pure thought. This is the process of thinking about an experience and reaching a conclusion about it without reference to the wider social reality. The religious type of terminology was carefully chosen since it allows for meditation, as well as the thought processes of the philosopher and the activities of the pure mathematician.

Reflective skills learning

This was called *reflective practice* in the book *Adult Learning in the Social Context* (Jarvis, 1987). It is one of the forms of learning that Schon (1983) concentrates upon, when he points out that professionals in practice think on their feet. In the process they often produce new skills as they respond to the uniqueness of their situation. Indeed, it was pointed out earlier that there are not many forms of skill that are learned in a totally unthinking manner, and so this may be regarded as a more sophisticated approach to learning practical subjects. It is not only learning a skill but learning about the knowledge undergirding the practice and, therefore, why the skill should be performed in a specific manner.

Experimental learning

This might have been called *reflective knowledge* in order to distinguish it from the previous form of learning. In this form of learning, theory is tried out in practice and the end-product of the experimentation is a form of knowledge that relates fully to the social reality of the practitioners. This approach to learning relates very closely to Kelly's (1963) understanding of human beings as scientists, seeking always to experiment on their environment.

It was pointed out above that these three forms of learning do not always have to be innovative, or change-orientated. It may be recalled that Argyris has two types of learning and in discussing these, he (1982 pp159–60) made this point:

> first is the misunderstanding that the goal of Model II implies that Model I is somehow bad or ineffective and should be suppressed.

On the contrary, Model I is the most appropriate theory in use for routine, programmed activities or emergency situations (such as rescuing survivors) that require prompt, unilateral action. We must not forget that the strategy of all organizations is to decompose double loop problems into single loop ones. The major part of everyday life learning in an organization is related to single loop learning. Double loop learning is crucial, because it allows us to examine and correct the way we are dealing with any issue and our underlying assumptions about it.

For Argyris, then, the more innovative forms of learning are crucial, but the other approaches are just as significant. While he employs the terms single and double loop, it is proposed to utilize the terms conformist and innovative reflective learning here. Both of these terms now need to be discussed. Botkin *et al.* (1979) employ the terms maintenance and innovative learning and these reflect the ideas contained here. It will be recalled that Freire (1972a, 1972b *inter alia*) recognized that there were two types of response in his forms of education: the one he called the 'banking concept of education' in which the learning was non-reflective, and the other he called 'problem posing education' in which he thought the learning would be innovative. However, Freire has not really constructed a full typology of learning and he has omitted some of the intermediate forms and, consequently, his problem posing education relates only in part to innovative reflective learning. In contrast, Habermas (1972) has three forms of learning: the technical, the practical and the emancipatory. His emancipatory form is similar to Freire's problem posing form of education, and not precisely the same as the innovatory reflective learning that is discussed here. The word innovatory is preferred to emancipatory because the connotations of this word are revolutionary and while innovation might be revolutionary, it does not have to be. Hence, the word seeks to convey change, rather than only revolutionary change.

Therefore, it may be seen that human beings do not merely receive a stimulus and respond to it: they have to think about it! Reflection is a significant element in human learning and one that it is important for teacher practitioners and preceptors to take into consideration in providing students with the opportunities to learn about aspects of their practical work. However, reflection itself is not a simple process that occurs automatically or only at one level. Mezirow (1981 p24) suggested that there are seven levels of reflectivity, although in his more recent writings he has moved away from concern for reflective thought:

1 *reflectivity*: awareness of seeing, thinking or acting
2 *affective reflectivity*: awareness of feelings

3 *discriminant reflectivity*: assessment of the efficiency of reflection in the context of reality
4 *judgmental reflectivity*: being aware of the subjective value judgments about reflections
5 *conceptual reflectivity*: assessment of whether the theoretical concepts employed are sufficient to explain perceived reality
6 *psychic reflectivity*: considering the adequacy of the evidence employed to explain perceived reality
7 *theoretical reflectivity*: awareness that taken-for-granted assumptions may be less than sufficient to explain perceived reality.

Mezirow suggested that the first four of these levels of reflectivity are of a lower order, which he regarded as 'consciousness', while the latter are regarded as 'critical-consciousness'. Becoming critically aware is an important stage in the development of any person, especially those being educated to enter social work, nursing, midwifery and health visiting. However, criticality is not sufficient and it is a precursor to creativity. As one of the main aims of education, teacher practitioners should strive to produce critically aware fellow practitioners who are able to be innovative about their practice when the conditions demand it, so long as that creativity is manifest within the bounds of safe practice, rather than recruits to the profession who merely conform to the theory and practice with which they are presented.

Teacher practitioners, mentors and preceptors are facilitating the experiences from which the learners and mentees learn, and if they are too authoritative in their actions they might well produce non-reflective learning outcomes. However, the facilitators' role is to provide a relatively safe environment whereby the learners can feel free enough to question the taken-for-granted knowledge and practices and be prepared to act differently in their practice. This situation enables them to produce their own repertoire of skills and their own bodies of knowledge which helps them in their own professional development. The way that teacher practitioners and mentors perform their role and create such a teaching and learning environment is vital to this process and, for instance, they should:

- be prepared to let the learners think things out for themselves
- ask sufficient, relevant questions to encourage the process of reflection
- allow the learners to think things through at their own pace
- not seem too anxious that the learners should actually reach a conclusion
- not expect that the learners will necessarily arrive at the same conclusion as they themselves have reached
- not pressurize the students to reject solutions with which they disagree.

By this approach, teacher practitioners and mentors demonstrate recognition of the adulthood and maturity of the learners and encourage autonomy and independence which are both essential attributes in the practice of social work, nursing, midwifery and health visiting.

ADULT LEARNING AND ANDRAGOGY

The concept of adulthood has exercised the minds of a number of writers on adult education, including Knowles (1980) and Paterson (1979). The intricacies of that discussion are not really the concern of this book, but it is very important to recognize that in the process of ageing the individual changes physiologically, psychologically and socially. Physiologically the body changes quite dramatically during this process, so that strength, reaction time, learning, vision, respiratory and circulatory functions all eventually undergo decline. Psychologically, the adult continues to develop, although no single classification of developmental stages is agreed upon by the scholars. Erikson's (1965) famous eight ages of man indicate four that are significant for all teachers of adults. If this is combined with Schaie's and Parr's thesis (1981) that there are three stages in intellectual development in adulthood – achievement, responsibility and reintegration – and only one in adolescence – acquisition – a table like Table 4.2 may be constructed.

Thus it may be seen that in different stages in the life cycle individuals have different orientations to learning and different perceptions of the self. Each of the experiences of life expand individuals' reservoir of knowledge and understanding, so that it is now claimed that crystallized intelligence, influenced by education and experience, expands between the ages of 19 and 61 years, whereas fluid intelligence, biologically-determined intellectual ability, declines during the same period (Cross, 1981 p162). These two changes may balance each other out, so that adults can continue to learn effectively throughout their working life, although the method of learning might well change significantly. Hence, it may be necessary to take these changes into consideration when developing an understanding and a theoretical perspective on adult learning. This is precisely what Knowles (1980) has attempted

Table 4.2 Adult development and learning

Age	Characteristics	Cognitive development
Adolescence	Ego identity versus Acquisition	Role diffusion
Early adulthood	Intimacy versus Achievement	Isolation
Middle adulthood	Generativity versus Responsibility	Stagnation
Late adulthood	Integrity versus Re-integration	Despair

to do in developing his well-known theory of andragogy – the art and science of helping adults learn. This theory has been demonstrated to be weak in recent years (Hartree, 1984; Tennant, 1986), and while Knowles' work grew out of a certain historical situation in the 1960s it does highlight a number of points that teacher practitioners and mentors might well wish to consider. In his original writings on andragogy, Knowles (1980 pp43–4) highlighted four significant assumptions:

- *the learner* moves from dependence to independence during maturation
- *the learner's experience* becomes an increasingly rich resource for learning
- *readiness to learn*: adults are ready to learn material relevant to their life situation
- *orientation to learning*: adults wish to apply what they learn, so that education should be organized around comprehensive categories.

In more recent writings he added two more characteristics: motivation of the adult (Knowles, 1984) and the need to know (Knowles, 1989). The fact that he can just add or subtract characteristics in this manner demonstrates clearly the lack of any carefully formulated theoretical foundations to andragogy. Indeed, Knowles himself has on occasions admitted that this is an approach that might be used with children, etc., but then continues to treat it as if it is an adult theory. Nursing and midwifery have certainly embraced andragogical perspectives without really enjoining the debate about its theoretical coherence and acceptability. Despite the many criticisms, however, the very persistence of the concept indicates that it embodies some truths that reflect the experiences of educators of adults. Hence, andragogy may indicate an ideology about teaching and learning with adults that may lead adult educators to produce an environment that enhances adults' learning processes. Most certainly these significant assumptions are relevant to the work of the teacher practitioner in the majority of situations.

COGNITIVE LEARNING STYLES

Earlier in this chapter it was suggested that some learners may be more effective if they start with a holistic perspective, and in the previous section it was indicated that as individuals age so their approaches to learning change. Hence, it may be recognized that different people have different styles of learning, something that it is important for teacher practitioners to ascertain with their own students. It is well known, for instance, that some people learn more effectively by reading, whilst others prefer to see or hear in order to maximize their acquisition of knowledge, etc. There have been a number of different formulations of learning styles (see Honey and Mumford, 1986; Kolb, 1984; Knox, 1977 pp447–9; Jarvis, 1983b pp83–7) and, since the teacher practitioner should be aware of these, some of the major ones are discussed briefly below.

- *Concrete versus Abstract*: Some learners like to start with the concrete situation such as experience, while others prefer to commence with an abstract, theoretical idea.
- *Converger versus Diverger*: The converger is best at abstract conceptualization and active experimentation and in situations where there is a single correct solution, whereas divergers are best at concrete experiences and reflective observation where they can generate ideas and have broad perspectives.
- *Focuser versus Scanner*: Focusers examine problems as a totality and generate hypotheses as a result of reflection that may be modified in the light of new information, whereas scanners select one aspect of the problem and assume it is the solution until subsequent information disproves it when they have to recommence the task.
- *Holistic versus Serialistic*: Some learners see a phenomenon as a whole while others prefer to string together the parts.
- *Impulsivity versus Reflectivity*: Some learners respond first and reflect later, while others reflect first and respond later.

Obviously learners adopt a variety of these types rather than functioning entirely in one of them. Indeed, Laschinger and Boss (1984) discovered that the majority of nurses in their research had concrete learning styles and that they were more influenced by people-orientated factors in their career choice. A later study (Laschinger, 1986) found that most nursing environments are predominantly concrete in learning orientation, which would be no surprise given the orientation to practical knowledge and practice itself which forms the basis of nursing.

Even so, learners might have preferred learning styles and it is useful to be aware of their most effective learning style, so that the teacher practitioners may prepare handouts for the student who learns best by reading, cassette tapes (especially for community nurses who have to drive between visits) or discussions for those who are more effective learners from audio input, etc. Additionally, the teacher practitioners and mentors may wish to present the whole situation to a holistic learner but not to a serialistic one, etc. Even though there has been a considerable amount of research on learning styles it is also important to recognize that 'there are only hints of association between cognitive style and learning effectiveness for adults' (Knox, 1977 p448). However, this may be, in part, because less research has actually been conducted with adults than with children in the learning situation. Another important reason for teacher practitioners knowing the preferred learning style of their students is because it may be necessary for them to help their students become more effective in some other styles which would be beneficial to their work situation.

LEARNING IN THE AFFECTIVE DOMAIN

The affective domain relates to the area of feelings and emotions and it is an aspect of teaching and learning that has received far less emphasis than the cognitive domain. However, it has been recognized in the education of adults that feelings may either enhance or inhibit adult learning, so that it is important to consider this particular aspect here. In addition, it is significant for the teacher practitioners and mentors to be aware of education in the affective domain because social work, nursing, midwifery and health visiting are concerned with the care of people, and it is necessary for practitioners to have attitudes that enhance the care that they provide. However, it is recognized that this is a very difficult area to explore and ideas like 'acceptable attitudes' are contentious. But their importance in the work of the teacher practitioner is such that they need consideration. This section explores first, the relationships between emotions and learning and, then, the recognition and teaching of attitudes.

EMOTIONS AND LEARNING

A considerable body of knowledge exists in the field of the education of adults about the relationship between feelings and learning, and reference to some of it has already been made in this chapter. Considerable emphasis has been placed upon the self-concept of the learner throughout this discussion since it is recognized that there are a number of factors in education that can and do prove stressful to the adult, such as fear that:

- the teaching and learning process will repeat some of the more unhappy experiences that the learners have had at school; this is true both for those who were successful in school and those who were less successful
- since the learners' role has not traditionally been associated with adulthood, it may conflict with their self-perception
- they may not have confidence to succeed because it is generally, but wrongly, thought that adults are not capable of learning new ideas.

Each of these points relates to the way in which adults are inhibited from learning and progressing because of a lack of belief in themselves. Belbin and Belbin (1972 p159) write:

Adults must believe in themselves as learners and each should be encouraged to relate this concept to the image of himself.

The greatest barrier to training arises from people believing that learning is not for them ... After discovering that they have learned, adults begin to see themselves as learners.

In the individualized teaching and learning situation, the teacher practitioners, preceptors and mentors are in a position to understand the students' perceptions of themselves and to structure their learning experiences in such a way as to ensure that they regard themselves as successful learners. The teacher practitioners and preceptors can, therefore:

- help the learners to respect themselves
- help the learners to realize that they are able to reflect upon their experiences and learn from them
- provide feedback to the learners so that they are able to become aware of what they have learned
- enhance the learners' self-image.

Hence, the teacher practitioners and other professionals working in an individualized teaching and learning situation are in a position to help the learners to feel more confident about learning which will almost certainly result in more consistent and effective learning. Rogers (1969; 1983; and Rogers and Freiberg, 1994) has argued most cogently that given a sense of freedom and confidence the most effective learning occurs.

LEARNING AND ATTITUDES

An attitude may be defined as 'an enduring system of positive or negative evaluations, emotional feelings and pro or con action tendencies with respect to a social object' (Krech, Crutchfield and Ballachey, 1962 p177), so that it may be seen that there is some similarity between attitudes and values.

Attitudes have both a cognitive and an affective element, and a behavioural tendency, so while teacher practitioners and mentors are able to observe students' behaviour in social work, nursing, midwifery or health visiting practice, and in interaction with both colleagues and patients, they can never be sure that the behaviour always reflects precisely what the students are thinking, or feeling. At the same time, consistent behavioural patterns may be more closely an expression of thoughts and feelings, and consistent patterns may actually illustrate the values that a student holds.

It may be recalled that Krathwohl (1964) devised a classification scheme for educational objectives in the affective domain: receiving, responding, valuing, organizing and characterizing a value or a value complex. Davies (1976 p156) suggested that this is not really a taxonomy of educational objectives but rather a continuum through which individuals pass from awareness to acceptance to preference of a particular value. Knowledge of such a continuum is important for teacher practitioners and preceptors who may be required to make students aware of other values than the ones that they currently display (for example, other ways of treating the elderly, the unkempt; other approaches to learning new knowledge, etc.). However, it would be indoctrination, rather than education, if the teacher practitioners deliberately set out with the intention of making the learners hold the same values that they themselves regard as professionally acceptable.

Nevertheless, there is a place for teaching values and, at least, giving students the opportunity to consider alternatives. Lewin and his associates (1952) investigated methods of doing this, comparing two different techniques: lecture followed by handout with group discussion. They discovered that group discussion was much more effective than the lecture in producing attitude change and, in a further study, they discovered that a group decision at the end of a discussion was more effective than individual instruction in producing changes. Hence, it appears that discussion is more effective than instruction in producing attitude change and groups are more effective than individuals. Therefore, the teacher practitioners and preceptors are at a disadvantage in not having a group of students if they consider that specific students should reconsider their attitude to any aspect of their work, although they can discuss it with the students and then leave it to them to reach their own conclusions.

LEARNING SKILLS

It will be recalled from the theory of learning discussed earlier in this chapter that there were two types of skills learning: the non-reflective and the reflective. Frequently, the teaching of skills has adopted the approach of non-reflective learning, so that students are expected to copy a demonstration, etc. However, it is suggested that there might be more than one correct way to perform some skills, and procedures and practitioners should be encouraged to consider the approach most acceptable to themselves, so long as it is safe and the outcomes acceptable.

Teaching psychomotor skills may form a significant element in the work of some teacher practitioners, so it is important to recognize that the same psychological and physiological aspects apply to this domain as they do to the cognitive. Indeed, it is important for the learner to recognize that age is no bar to learning to perform a psychomotor skill at speed: Belbin and Belbin (1972) document the fact that older people can learn skills even if the learning process might be a little more difficult than it is with teenagers. However, the significant point is that new techniques can be learned by older people, especially if they have ample opportunity to practise them at their own pace in private, and perhaps upon a dummy. However, it must also be recognized that there are problems for adults when they are learning skills. For instance, Smith (1977 p198) writes:

> Various authors have found that older trainees have less confidence, take longer to learn and find it difficult to eliminate the mistakes that they are making ... in addition, the older trainee may be unduly quality conscious, which inhibits the building of skills that depend on speed of action.

Despite this depressing picture, Smith suggests that this actually reflects the method of training rather than the acquisition of new skills. He points out that the discovery method, whereby the trainees actually discover the relevant principles and relationships for themselves, is one that enables the older person to acquire relevant skills. However, there are a number of obvious problems about the discovery method in nursing, midwifery and health visiting that need further discussion (see Chapter 5).

In Chapter 3 the educational objectives in skills training were discussed and two sets of objectives produced. Harrow's (1972) developmental taxonomy relates to maturation, but Simpson's (1966) approach outlines various aspects of learning and then proceeds through the stages of the acquisition of a complicated skill leading to its performance in an automatic manner. Clearly automatic behaviour occurs only after practice and this will itself occur only when learners have the confidence and the supportive environment in which to undertake it. Hence, the teacher practitioners' and mentors' role may again lie in the creation of a supportive environment in which the students are given the confidence to practise. The teacher practitioners' and preceptors' role is, therefore, a very skilled one embracing knowledge, skill and sensitivity through which the learners feel free to practise and to experiment. However, one of the topics of Chapter 5 is teaching techniques, but before these are discussed it may prove useful to summarize the principles of adult learning discussed in this chapter.

LEARNING HOW TO LEARN

In recent years the idea of learning how to learn has come to the forefront of the concerns of work-based learning. Indeed, it is a core skill for many. A major part of the role of mentors, preceptors and teacher practitioners is helping their mentees or students to learn from their experiences in the workplace. Smith (1982) highlighted the various approaches to this, many of which are concerned with teaching and are covered in Chapter 5. At the same time, it is important that facilitators of work-based learning see their role as not just being teachers but also of making students aware of the significance of learning from their experiences and of showing them ways of utilizing the wide variety of resources that are available to them to continue their professional development on their own initiative.

Conclusion

This chapter has provided a broad overview of some of the important elements of the complex processes of learning and they are summarized as follows.

There are at least three learning responses:

- non-learning responses to experience
- non-reflective responses to experience – these are ones which are often regarded as the core of learning
- reflective approaches to learning – these actually form the basis for reflective practice.

Adults are:

- able to learn throughout the greater part of their lifespan, so that attention has to be paid to the method of learning as well as the content of what is learned
- continuing to develop and mature so that the reasons why they wish to learn are significant to the process
- facilitated to learn through the provision of experiences which provoke a need to question
- always acquiring experiences which are a rich resource for further learning
- able to learn more effectively when the relevance of what is being learned is recognized
- less able to learn effectively when placed in a stress-creating situation.

In the teaching and learning interaction, adults:

- should always be treated with dignity and humanity
- should learn in a pleasurable environment
- will learn more effectively if correct learning is rewarded by positive reinforcement
- will learn more effectively if they have self-confidence

- will learn more effectively if they are free to work at their own pace.

Traditionally theories of learning underplay:

- the humanity of the learners
- the experience of the adult learners
- the place of reflection in the learning process.

Reflection in the adult learning process:

- should be facilitated
- may involve either a conscious or a critically conscious appraisal of the experience and lead to a creative or innovative outcome where appropriate
- may develop independence of mind and action.

Attitudes and values are:

- learned in precisely the same way as other types of learning
- important for practice.

Skills may be learned by adults through:

- discovery methods
- learning individual stages in a sequence.

Hence it may be seen that adults are able to learn throughout most of their lives and that the manner by which the learning process is facilitated may enhance or inhibit the learning. Therefore, the role of the teachers of adults is quite crucial to this process and Chapter 5 examines teaching and learning strategies appropriate for adults in an individualized teaching and learning situation.

Teaching adults in individualized teaching and learning

5

This chapter explores:
- *The relationship between theory and practice*
- *Teaching styles and models of teaching*
- *Teaching methods for individualized teaching and learning*
- *Some other teaching methods*
- *Teaching aids*
- *Preparing a teaching and learning session.*

INTRODUCTION

Teaching is perhaps one of the most widely practised activities in the world: parents teach their children; children teach their parents; adults teach adults in everyday social interaction; teachers teach pupils, etc. In everyday conversation individuals disseminate information and other people learn from it: the latter are, therefore, taught by the former. Hence, it could legitimately be claimed that during every individuals's lifetime they will perform the function of teacher on many occasions. However, they will not necessarily be accorded the status of teacher unless they hold a designated role as one, the reason being that the status of teacher is usually restricted to those persons who perform the occupational role of teacher within an educational institution and who usually gain financial reward for teaching students or pupils.

But teaching obviously occurs in contexts other than that of the formal school or college, so that it might be possible to classify teaching in some way according to the type of situation in which it occurs. For instance, parents teach children in an informal context, so that the educational process maybe regarded as informal and the teaching viewed as being within the *informal mode*. By contrast, teachers teach their pupils within the formal structure of the school or college, so that formal education and the teaching may be seen to fall within a *formal mode*. However, neither of these two types are actually applicable to the situation in which teacher practitioners teach their students or mentors help their mentees. Clearly there is a third approach. Recently the concept of *non-formal education* has been introduced into the world of education and Coombes and Ahmed (1974) define this as:

> any organized, systematic, educational activity carried on outside the framework of the formal system to provide selected types of learning to particular sub-groups in the population, adults as well as children. (cited in La Belle 1982 pp161–2)

This type of education obviously falls between the two previous categories mentioned, but the above definition does not correlate exactly with the work of teacher practitioners or preceptors since they perform their role outside the formal classroom but within the formal system of professional education. Hence, it is possible to adapt this definition slightly and to suggest that non-formal teaching is 'any organized, systematic, educational activity conducted outside the formal context of the classroom to provide selected types of learning to particular sub-groups in the population, adults as well as children'. Thus it may be claimed that within this definitional framework the teacher practitioner's role may be regarded as a non-formal teaching one. Such an approach has been developed by Srinivasan (1977) within the context of adult learning.

The above definition does not specify what is taught by the teacher practitioners, or anyone else occupying a similar role, in the context of non-formal education, and this is significant because there is often a division made between teaching theory in the formal classroom situation and teaching skills in the non-formal context of professional practice. Hence, teacher practitioners and preceptors are sometimes regarded as 'only a teacher of skills'. Such a derogatory categorization, as implied by this remark, fails to do justice to their role nor does it show awareness of the inter-relationship between theory and practice. Nor does such a stance take cognisance of the students' needs. For example, the study conducted by Ogier in 1974 (cited in Davis, 1983) shows that learner nurses expected ward sisters to teach them the theory relating to the skills that they were being taught. The sisters, who were rated most highly by the learners, related theory to practice on an individualized teaching and learning basis, especially if that teaching is undertaken with enthusiasm (Van Hoozer, 1987). Hence, this chapter commences with a discussion about this relationship and, thereafter, it explores various styles, methods and aids in teaching.

THE RELATIONSHIP BETWEEN THEORY AND PRACTICE

In an earlier chapter it was stated that those teachers who teach theoretical knowledge are ascribed a higher status than those of whom it is claimed teach only skills. It is maintained here, however, that this discussion is over-simplistic and that this status differential is one that reflects a misleading philosophical ideal. Indeed, teacher practitioners, mentors and preceptors might be teachers of both theory and practice because of the nature of their interrelationships.

The Greeks had the idea that the educated man, always 'man' in their culture (!), was one whose life was based upon continual contemplation, for by so doing argued Aristotle the product is a rational individual who both performs good actions and is happy. Hence, for Aristotle:

> man's actions were performed as a result of rational consideration prior to the act. Ever since that time thinkers have been 'predisposed to find that it was in their capacity for rigorous theory that lay the superiority of man over animals, of civilized men over barbarious, and even of the divine mind over human minds.' (Ryle, 1949 p27).

Hence, 'to know that' has traditionally been distinguished from 'to know how' and theoretical knowledge been accorded higher status than practical knowledge. Indeed, Ryle (1949 p28) claimed:

> Theorists have been so preoccupied with the task of investigating the nature, the source, and the credentials of the theories that we adopt that they have for the most part ignored the question what it is for someone to know how to perform tasks. In ordinary life, on the contrary, as well as in the special business of teaching, we are much more concerned with people's competences than with their cognitive repertoires, with the operations than with the truths that they learn.

Ryle's claims in the above passage are perfectly understandable and reflect a realistic analysis of the current situation, and thinking about 'knowledge how' a task should be performed has been a much neglected activity. However, his analysis of this activity led him to make the following claim (1949 p32), that:

> When I do something intelligently, i.e. thinking what I am doing, I am doing one thing and not two. My performance has a special procedure or manner, not special antecedents.

Such a conclusion may be considered extreme and may not be universally acceptable since it is too behaviouristic, but one of the major merits of this position is that it focuses attention upon the knowledge necessary to undertake the performance of a skill, and this was discussed quite fully in Chapter 1. However, it will be claimed here that 'being able' and 'knowledge how' can be learned simultaneously in practice situations, since it involves two learning processes.

But in the course of his discussion, Ryle also suggested, for instance, that a person does not have to know the nature of logic before arguing logically, so that 'knowledge that' does not have to precede 'knowledge how' to do so. This is a position that was indicated in Chapter 4, when it was suggested that adults might learn psychomotor skills best by first being given the opportunity to explore the relevant principles and relationships for themselves, so that when they begin to practise they are not functioning in total ignorance and, indeed, the actions become more meaningful so that they can begin to theorize from practice much more quickly. Thereafter, they can acquire both the 'knowledge how' and, more significantly, the 'knowledge that' it happens. Perhaps, this argument could be extended even further, in accord with the learning processes discussed earlier, and it might be shown that 'knowledge why' may be developed logically from reflective practice. Hence, it may be claimed that in the learning process, 'knowledge how' may most effectively occur first and, indeed, it might be claimed that in many areas of human behaviour it actually occurs automatically first in any case. But it is maintained here that the processes and types of knowledge and action are different so that Ryle's argument is in no way accepted here.

Why, then, does it appear that 'knowing how' and 'knowing that' are fused into a single process in intelligent action? Perhaps this occurs because the different forms of knowledge may not occur with the same intensity in intelligent behaviour because much of the process appears to be taken for granted in habitualized actions. Berger and Luckmann (1967 p71) refer to this process as habitualization:

> Habitualized actions, of course, retain their meaningful character for the individual although the meanings involved become embedded as routines in his [sic] general stock of knowledge, taken for granted by him and at hand for his future projects. Habitualization carries with it an important psychological gain that choices are narrowed. While in theory there are a hundred ways to go about a project of building a canoe out of matchsticks, habitualization narrows the choice to one. This frees the individual from 'all those decisions,' providing a psychological relief that has its basis in man's undirected instinctual structure.

Berger and Luckmann are pointing to the significant inter-relationship of 'knowledge how' and 'knowledge that' and in some instances, 'knowledge why'. They are not claiming that intelligent acts of skill do not have any thought, only that individuals having internalized the knowledge and having habitualized the skills are able to perform procedures without having to think greatly about them. Indeed, this is the traditional goal of a great deal of training! In the course of their duties nurses, midwives and health visitors perform many habitualized actions (for example, aseptic dressing technique, recording blood pressure, vision testing, etc.), but performing in such a manner can be very dangerous, since practitioners might miss little tell-tale signs.

In addition, when situations arise where the internalized knowledge and the habitualized procedure are not directly applicable to the situation, the actors have either to change their course of action or utilize another procedure that fits most closely the new situation. Merely experimenting with different established procedures is rather bureaucratic and not necessarily a sound basis of professional practice, so that teacher practitioners and preceptors might encourage their learners to utilize their knowledge (both 'that' and 'why') in order to develop a new course of action. Hence, there is a sense in which theory and practice come together in an active manner when professional practitioners have to solve a problem in the process of implementing care.

Figure 5.1 illustrates clearly an inter-relationship between theory and practice which implies that to separate them in any way would impoverish both. Ryle was clearly right in seeking to discredit the over-emphasis placed upon theory but he does not appear correct in suggesting that intelligent activity is a single act. But theory and practice are closely inter-related, so that it would be quite false to regard teacher practitioners or preceptors as 'only teachers of skills'. They have to help the students by combining the two, so that they can both utilize internalized knowledge and habitualized skills in developing problem-solving techniques as appropriate.

In precisely the same way teacher practitioners and preceptors need to have a theoretical knowledge of education so that they can

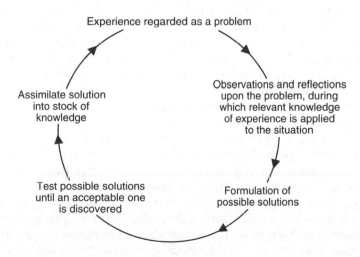

Figure 5.1 A problem-solving cycle

undertake their role as a teacher. Hence, earlier in this book the problems for the teacher practitioners and preceptors, as having two professionalisms, were discussed, and the remainder of this chapter concentrates upon some theoretical and practical approaches to the teaching aspect of their role.

TEACHING STYLES AND MODELS OF TEACHING

Non-formal teaching in individualized teaching and learning is not a stereotypical process, and teacher practitioners, mentors and preceptors may all adopt different approaches to the performance of their teaching role. These different approaches may be similar in many ways to those adopted by a teacher in a more formal teaching role. For instance, teacher practitioners and preceptors may be authoritarian, democratic or *laissez-faire*; they may regard their students as highly motivated or inherently lazy, who have to be cajoled or coerced into activity; they may see their role as implanting knowledge or in providing opportunities for students to learn. These different approaches have usually been referred to as teaching styles, but they actually reflect different approaches and models to teaching itself, so they will be discussed here and this will lead into an explanation of the nature of teaching itself.

In the 1930s Kurt Lewin and his associates (Lippitt and White, 1958) undertook some research into different leadership styles, highlighting three approaches: authoritarian, democratic and *laissez-faire*. While this research was conducted with ten-year-old boys in group situations at youth camps and, consequently, far removed from the situation of the teacher practitioner, it is mentioned here because there is a sense in which teachers assume a leadership role. In the teaching and learning interaction it is quite possible for teacher practitioners and mentors to be authoritarian, democratic or even *laissez-faire*, although this final approach is less likely by virtue of the situation. Teacher practitioners and preceptors may be authoritarian – stern, bossy, seeking always to tell and direct their learners. By contrast, they may wish to do very little and let the students 'get on with it' or merely to watch them perform. Lewin and his associates discovered that while the authoritarian leaders appeared to get a lot of work completed as a result of a high level of activity, it only occurred during their presence since they had not really made the participants feel that the work was their own. The *laissez-faire* leaders achieved very little, whether they were present or not. By contrast, Lewin and his associates discovered that democratic leaders were able to achieve co-operation from the children who then worked well together on their projects whether they were present or absent from the situation, since they had decided upon what to do together and it was therefore their own work. This approach is clearly more in accord with the perspective adopted in this book and reflects the humanistic interaction between teacher practitioner and learner discussed in earlier chapters.

According to Davies (1971), teachers are also managers of the teaching and learning situation. McGregor (1960) highlighted two different approaches to management that have some relevance here: he called these Theory X and Theory Y. The former suggests that managers regard individuals as having to be cajoled or coerced into activity by threat of punishment or by promise of reward because they regard people as fundamentally lazy. This is sometimes referred to as the 'carrot-and-stick' approach. By contrast, the latter theory starts from the pre-supposition that human beings are self-motivated and seek to fulfil their potential. Similarity may be seen here between this management theory and the leadership research by Lewin and his associates, since Theory Y reflects a philosophy similar to that inherent in democratic leadership and is in harmony with the approach that is highlighted throughout this study, reflecting a humanistic philosophy.

Both of the previous two processes have indicated that an ideological perspective will result in a style of leadership or management that is relevant to teacher practitioners, mentors and preceptors as they consider how to perform their role. However, these approaches have not actually been about teaching *per se* and it is perhaps significant to note that no simple association of philosophy and the actual style of teaching can be drawn in this manner.

Other writers have suggested other styles. Van Hoozer (1987), for instance, suggests that there are four styles: telling, selling, participating and delegating. In another approach, Nouwen (1971) suggested that there are *violent teachers*, who are seen as competitive and dominant and who alientate the students, and there are *redemptive teachers* who work with the students to draw out each other's potential in an open situation. Another approach to teaching styles has been that of Fox (1983) who also has four types:

1 *Transfer*: teachers treat knowledge as a commodity to be transferred to the students
2 *Shaping*: teachers seek to mould students to a predetermined pattern
3 *Travelling*: teachers are the expert guides on the educational journey
4 *Growing*: the learning process is one in which the students grow and develop.

Each of these approaches offers different interpretations of the style in which teachers perform their roles. Jarvis (1995a) has also suggested three different approaches to teaching, which are didactic, socratic and facilitative; these are both styles and categories of teaching methods, and in the latter context they will form the basis for the discussion on methods. However, they are first elaborated briefly here as teaching styles. Didactic teaching assumes that teachers have knowledge to impart and that they adopt the style of 'giving out' their knowledge to the student. The socratic approach, however, assumes that the students are not empty receptacles to be filled but rather active thinkers so that the teachers' style becomes more questioning, requiring the learners to become problem-solvers and more reflective. Hence, the teachers are now seeking to draw out rather than put into the students. Facilitative teaching is a style whereby the teacher steps back from the actual learning process, having first provided the conditions in which learning can actually occur, but they are available as resources if the students require advice or guidance.

Clearly, it may be seen that authoritarian leaders may be more likely to be didactic or violent teachers, but the contrast may not necessarily be true. Similarly, democratic leaders are more likely to be socratic and redemptive travelling companions, but this need not necessarily occur. Someone who holds the ideology of Theory Y may well practise a variety of these teaching styles on different occasions. Hence, there is no simple association between all the styles discussed in this section even though it is easy to see some of the associations that might arise. However, from all the discussion it may be seen that there are fundamentally two models of teaching:

1 *a teacher-centred model*, in which the teacher decides, the teacher controls and the teacher imparts knowledge
2 *a learner-centred model*, in which the learner is involved in the decision-making process in a democratic manner and the learner's acquisition of knowledge, skill and attitude is more significant than the teacher's activity.

Consequently, it may be asked 'What is teaching?' If teaching is not the impartation of knowledge, as is often assumed, what is it? Perhaps teaching might best be defined as the process of helping others learn. This, then, is the activity in which teacher practitioners, mentors and preceptors are involved and it is now necessary to explore some of the methods by which they might perform this activity.

TEACHING METHODS FOR INDIVIDUALIZED TEACHING AND LEARNING

All learning stems from experience. Perhaps that was one of the most important implications from the experiential learning process that was discussed earlier, so that the experience of working in the professional situation is perhaps the greatest single learning experience that can be provided for students. Nevertheless, it is the job of teacher practitioners and preceptors to ensure that the experiences provided are fully utilized and that the lessons that can be learned from them are learned efficiently and correctly, so that they need to be competent in the use of the non-formal techniques which are applicable to the individualized teaching and learning situation. In this section several types are discussed: demonstration; talk; discussion; role play and simulation; case study; practical assignments; visits and trips. These six techniques form an approximate continuum from teacher-centred to learner-centred models of teaching, although in the ensuing discussion it will be seen that even the more teacher-centred approaches may be utilized in a learner-centred manner.

DEMONSTRATION

Demonstrating a psychomotor skill is often regarded as the method whereby learners acquire knowledge of how to perform from an expert. Having witnessed an expert performance, learners are then expected to practise until they are as proficient as the demonstrator. This approach has been generally regarded as not having been very successful with older learners so that, according to Belbin and Belbin (1972), it has become general practice to recruit only younger people to some occupations that require manual dexterity. However, Belbin and Belbin (1972 pp44–5) suggest that if a skill is broken down into its component parts and that each stage is demonstrated and practised slowly and only gradually is the whole procedure unified, it is possible for older learners to acquire new skills fairly rapidly. They recognize, however, that one of the most difficult elements in this approach is that of learning each stage of the skill slowly and precisely in the first instance and only, subsequently, when the procedure is learned, should it be speeded up.

Following this approach, it would prove useful for teacher practitioners and preceptors to analyze carefully the skills that they are required to teach and sub-divide them into discrete stages, so that in the individualized teaching and learning situation they can help the students with each of the component parts. In this way, the teacher practitioners and preceptors may help the learners acquire proficiency and fluency in skills and procedures more efficiently. It might be beneficial for teacher practitioners and preceptors to endeavour to undertake such an analysis whilst observing another practitioner performing that specific procedure.

Another factor that the teacher practitioners should consider when employing the demonstration method is whether the learners use the same hand as they do. For instance, if a teacher practitioner is right-handed and the learner left-handed, then she sees a different image of the practice than would her right-handed colleague. Hence, if teacher practitioners and preceptors work with the same hands as their learners, then the latter might be best positioned next to them but, when they use opposite hands, the learners should be placed directly facing them.

Teachers who are well-practised in a skill may sometimes forget the problems that they experienced in acquiring it and find it hard to empathize with students having difficulties. However, the teachers' style and ideology should be such that they endeavour always to reach out to the students and be with them as they undergo the difficulties of learning – being with them, in this sense, communicates non-verbally the care and concern that teachers should have for their students.

During the demonstration the teacher practitioners and preceptors should be aware of the taxonomies of objectives in the psychomotor domain discussed by Simpson and Harrow, mentioned in Chapter 3. However, even if the aforementioned facts are taken into consideration, a major weakness in the demonstration method is that the teacher practitioners and preceptors become role models, but their own way of proceeding may not actually be the most effective way for the students whom they are teaching to perform it. There may be other, even more effective, ways!

However, breaking down a procedure into its component parts is not as simple as it sounds, since Dreyfus and Dreyfus (1981, cited in de Tornyay and Thompson, 1982 p61) suggest that experts may have incorporated the various stages of the skill into their performance so that they are unable to identify the component parts. This is also a point that Nyiri (1988) makes when he points out that a great deal of practical knowledge is tacit so that experts might not necessarily be able to articulate that knowledge. It is for this reason that teacher practitioners and preceptors should observe someone else performing the procedure in order to break it down into its component parts. In addition, learners might seek to emulate the expert on occasions. In defence of apprenticeship, Polyani (1958 p53) wrote:

> To learn by example is to submit to authority . . . By watching the master and emulating his efforts in the presence of his example, the apprentice unconsciously picks up the rules of the art, including those which are not explicitly known to the master himself. Those hidden rules can be assimilated only by a person who surrenders himself to that extent uncritically to the imitation of another. A society which wants to preserve a fund of personal knowledge must submit to tradition.

Teacher practitioners, mentors and preceptors might be regarded by their learners as experts simply because they are often the only experienced practitioners that the learners observe on a regular basis, so that they should always be aware that they might actually be regarded as expert role models by those with whom they work and whom they teach.

By contrast to this approach, which is a teacher-centred method, learner-centred discovery methods of learning skills are now regarded as more efficient. Smith (1977 p199) writes:

> In essence, the discovery method is a style of teaching which structures a situation so that the trainee learns by activity finding out the principles and relationships himself. Thus, for example, instead of a trainee being shown a piece of equipment and given a lecture on how it works, the trainee would be given the actual piece of equipment with the parts clearly labelled. Provided that safety considerations are taken into account, the trainee learns the function of each part and how the equipment works by operating it himself.

In this approach, teacher practitioners and preceptors facilitate the learning situation and thus allow the learners to work at their own pace; they encourage the students to master the equipment when they are ready, acting as motivators and helpers to the reflective process. Obviously this technique can be utilized quite easily for much of the equipment that student nurses and midwives are expected to employ in a hospital and even in the community, but where there are nursing and interpersonal skills that directly involve patients or clients this may make this particular technique inappropriate. In some instances, however, it might be possible for students to practise skills on a dummy in a training and learning ward or even on peers, prior to practising on patients/clients, so that where this is possible the discovery method may still be used. Practising on peers, however, has ethical implications that need to be taken into account before it is introduced. When employing the demonstration technique, teacher practitioners and preceptors should not be too unrealistic in their expectations of students' performances, but they should seek to ensure that the latter are safe to practise before allowing them to do so when they are unsupervised. Proficient performance may take a considerable time to achieve. Indeed, Benner (1984 p25) suggests that competency might only be achieved by nurses who have been in the same situations for two or three years, so that teacher practitioners and preceptors should always be aware of the progress that students make – however little it might appear – and commend them for it, since positive feedback is always an encouragement to continue learning. However, there are skills mostly of the interpersonal kind, that may not always be learned by the discovery method and therefore more appropriate techniques should be employed.

THE TALK

The talk is rather like a lecture, where teacher practitioners or preceptors address the students in a more formal manner and when the flow
of conversation is mainly from the teachers to the students. Giving information to the students in this manner may have a place in the work of
the teacher practitioners and preceptors, but they should be aware that
this technique is generally regarded as having limited value, especially
in teaching adults. Concentration spans vary: Trenaman (1951) claimed
that after 15 minutes the talk becomes an ineffective mode of communication, while Legge (1974 p59) implies that for some people from four
to five minutes is the maximum time that they can concentrate.
However, the talk is considered a relatively easy teaching technique, so
it is frequently employed, but if it is to be used by teacher practitioners
and preceptors then they should be aware of its limitations.

Even so, talks are often given and frequently expected, so it is important that teacher practitioners and preceptors acquire the skills of both
preparation and presentation. Talks do need careful and thorough
preparation, so that the listeners can follow the flow and logic of the
argument. Therefore, the structure of the talk is vital, almost as important as the content, for good content has no value if the listeners cannot
learn it! It is wise in a short talk to have no more than two or three
main points, each of which should flow logically from the other and, in
addition, it is useful to have both an introduction and a conclusion. The
old maxim has much validity: 'First, I tells 'em what I'm going to tell
'em, then I tells 'em and then I tells 'em what I've told 'em'. It is useful
for listeners to know what they are about to learn, so that they can
prepare their minds for it and it is beneficial to learning to help the
recipient of information itemize the main points at the end. Hence, one
simple structure for a talk might be:

1   *Introduction*, in which the rationale behind the presentation and the
    sequence of the main points is given
2   *Part I, Part II, Part III*, main body of information developed logically
    in a number of points (not necessarily three)
3   *Conclusion*, recapitulating the main points and summarizing the argu-
    ment.

It is always useful to prepare a talk very thoroughly, and often the
shorter the talk the more difficult it is to prepare because of the need
to condense material, so it may be necessary to spend longer planning
a five-minute address than a 15-minute talk. Many people find it very
useful to write out the whole talk during preparation rather than merely
sketching an outline, and such thoroughness in preparation is recommended, especially in the early days of a teaching career. In addition,

it is necessary to ensure that the language used bridges the gap between the expert teacher and the students who might not yet have acquired a professional vocabulary. Learners also find it more interesting for the talk to have practical applications, and relevance often counter-balances any weakness in presentation. When the talk is prepared, it may be useful to précis it for presentation purposes, for example, using just paragraph headings on a single sheet of paper, or on postcards.

When giving a talk, even to just one student, it is necessary to ensure that, wherever possible, the physical environment is conducive to learning. For instance, the place where the talk is given should be free from constant interruptions, the furniture should be comfortable and the teachers should sit in a position whereby they can maintain eye contact with the students in order to assess the extent to which they are understanding what is being presented to them. Sheets of paper and full notes may also be a hindrance to maintaining eye contact, so it is preferable to deliver a talk either without notes or, if this proves difficult, with as few as possible. In this manner the teacher practitioners and preceptors will have sufficient support to give them confidence, enough material to allow them to recreate their points and not too many notes to prevent eye contact with the students. Some teachers may be able to commit their whole talk to memory, which is good, provided that their address is not a recitation of what they have memorized but a recreation in a living setting.

During delivery, speech should be clear, words carefully articulated, especially since some people, with less than perfect hearing, are prone to accept that they have not always heard every word and interrupt and ask the teacher to repeat what she has said.

Even so, the limitations of this teaching technique have to be recognized and there are other methods, less teacher-centred, that teacher practitioners might employ. In some instances, guided reading could replace the talk and this might be followed by a discussion.

DISCUSSION METHODS

Discussion may appear to be a more natural approach to adopt in individualized teaching and learning than the rather stereotypical talk. Discussions are most useful in problem-posing and problem-solving approaches to teaching. There are basically three types of discussion method that may be utilized: teacher-controlled, guided and student-controlled.

Teacher-controlled discussion

In teacher-controlled discussion the teachers are still in charge of the interaction and they present the topic selected for discussion, but unlike the talk, they expect some verbal participation from the students; either by responding to questions, commenting on points or issues raised and by asking the teachers questions. Nevertheless, it is the teachers who direct the discussion, control its pace and often it is they who have selected the topic which is under consideration. Teacher practitioners and preceptors may find that this technique is more appropriate in the individualized teaching and learning situation in which they perform this role. As the teachers are controlling the interaction, it is important that their preparation is thorough and they may well undertake similar preparation to that described for the talk, but, in addition, they may work out the points where they would like, or expect, student participation. Clearly this approach has a number of advantages over the talk, including the fact that there is: student participation; active learning; less chance of the student losing concentration; opportunity for the students to discuss and even to disagree with the teachers; opportunity for the student to share relevant experiences; less artificiality in the non-formal teaching situation.

Guided discussion

Guided discussion is an approach that utilizes the students' experiences much more than controlled discussion. In this instance, the teachers seek to elicit information, knowledge, ideas, etc. from the students by a carefully prepared process of questioning. This is the socratic style, which was discussed earlier in the chapter, whereby the teachers endeavour to lead the students from what they already know into new realms of thought by building one question upon another, taking the students through a logical sequence of stages until they are able to draw conclusions or express new ideas. Because the teachers are utilizing the students' knowledge and building upon their answers, there could be a temptation to assume that the approach demands less preparation, but this is not so! In preparation, the teachers have to anticipate the students' response and endeavour to work out notes from those responses in order to ensure that the aims and objectives of the session are achieved. In addition, the teachers require a sound knowledge of the subject since the students' responses may make considerable demands upon the teachers' professional expertise.

Asking questions is an art (Bateman, 1990), one that the teacher practitioners should acquire in order to ensure that the learners are able to demonstrate their knowledge. Additionally, skilled questioning techniques can only enhance professional practice. Questions are asked for various reasons, for example, to obtain information, to stimulate reflection and creative thought, to assess learning outcomes, to determine learning needs, to clarify a situation, to establish and maintain social interaction. Obviously the purpose of the question will influence the way in which it is formulated and posed. Both the formulation and the manner in which it is asked will affect the response, and inexperienced teacher practitioners and preceptors often fail to get the type of reply that they seek from questions.

Questions may be classified in a variety of ways. De Tornyay and Thompson (1982 pp65–72) categorize them as follows:

- factual or descriptive
- clarifying
- higher order
- convergent and divergent.

Each of these is now briefly considered.

Factual or descriptive questions

These usually begin with: what, why, how, who, when or where. These questions elicit factual information which a person has memorized, a description of an event, situation, object or person. Questions of this type are:

- What factors contribute to hypothermia in the elderly?
- How is John's ulcer today?
- What foods contain calciferol?

These are the types of question that the teacher practitioners and preceptors should employ to ensure that the students actually have the 'knowledge that' and if appropriate has observed accurately the client or patient.

Clarifying questions

One of the purposes of clarifying questions is to enable the learners to elaborate upon an initial response or to help them reflect upon a learning situation. This may be undertaken by:

- seeking more information and/or additional meaning
- requiring justification of a previous response
- focusing the student's attention on a related issue
- prompting
- redirecting attention.

Higher order questions

These questions are more demanding than the previous types since they cannot be answered by memory recall, description or perception. They ask students to think and to learn from a previous experience and, as such, it may be seen that they are the type of question that teacher practitioners and preceptors should use to help the learner reflect upon an earlier learning experience. According to de Tornyay and Thompson (1982 p68) higher order questions perform three specific functions, as the following examples show:

- *evaluation*, for example, What were the priorities which led you to organize your caseload in this way today?
- *inferences*, for example, What did you learn about that nursing problem as a result of caring for Mrs Smith?
- *comparisons*, for example, What is the relationship between social class and perinatal mortality?

Convergent and divergent questions

In contrast to the above, some questions may be posed that encourage the 'intellectually convergent' or the 'intellectually divergent' to utilize their own orientation to thinking and learning. In the convergent mode, the students are encouraged to comprehend the task in hand and to focus closely upon it, whereas in the divergent approach the learners are given the opportunity to think more widely and to apply knowledge to a variety of situations in order to synthesize ideas, perceive relationships and to engage in creative problem solving.

Questions may appear threatening to students who have not been exposed to the socratic method of teaching, so that they should always be asked in a warm and friendly manner. Hence, it may be seen from the above discussion that both the type of question and the technique employed to pose it are pertinent to teaching and learning, so that it may be useful for teacher practitioners to practise this art.

Student-controlled discussion

Unlike the previous two approaches, student-controlled discussion allows the students to ask all the questions. Obviously, the degree to which students feel free to ask significant questions will depend upon the rapport that exists between the teacher practitioners or preceptors and the students. If, for instance, the students are being continuously assessed and they know that the teacher practitioners or preceptors are their assessors as well as their teachers, they may never feel able to ask such questions since they might feel that they would reveal their weaknesses rather than their strengths of having an enquiring mind, endeavouring to understand everything relevant to their professional practice. Hence, students should always be given the opportunity and encouraged to raise significant and searching questions about both professional practice and the manner in which the teacher practitioners or preceptors perform their dual role of teacher and professional practitioner. In other words, the teacher practitioners' and preceptors' professional knowledge, skills and attitudes should always be open to the student's searching enquiry. The students should be encouraged to ask questions by the teacher practitioners and the answers that they receive should always be honest. Hence, if the teachers or preceptors do not know the answer to a question, they should admit to it and thus suggest that they both endeavour to discover an answer. Such an approach facilitates active learning for both teachers and students. But will not the teacher practitioners or preceptors lose face with the student? Few people expect the teacher practitioners or preceptors to know everything, so provided this response is not forthcoming too frequently, it will do no harm to their reputation. Even so, teacher practitioners and preceptors may not actually always wish to answer questions that students ask, they may wish to respond with a further question, which leads the students into further realms of knowledge. Effective teachers do not always lead students from answer to answer, but often from one question to another.

While discussion methods may appear to be a little more time-consuming, they are approaches which the teacher practitioners and preceptors might wish to adopt since they allow them to be sure that the students have actually learned the knowledge and that they are also able to express what they know. Additionally, the guided discussion technique is useful to help students reflect upon their learning experiences, enabling them to capitalize upon their learning and to pursue more thoroughly the ideas that the experiences set in motion. Hence, they are beneficial techniques to be employed in individualized teaching and learning.

ROLE PLAY AND SIMULATION

These teaching and learning methods are basically the dramatization of 'real life' events in which the role players enact the roles which either they themselves, or others, would perform in the actual situation. The primary purpose is to enable the learners to experience, in a more protected environment, the emotions and the problems of people in everyday living. Clearly it has a number of uses in professional education, some of which will be referred to below. Role play is frequently unscripted but carefully prepared before the event, whereas simulation is the creation of an actual situation in which the procedures are far less spontaneous and are often played out over a longer period of time than role play.

There are many advantages in using these techniques because not only do they involve the students in active learning, but that learning is of an affective nature in which it is important for practitioners to consider their interpersonal skills, often in very stressful situations. This approach to their preparation, therefore, enables them to focus upon quite specific incidents and skills.

Role play can be employed to help students experience a specific role prior to having to perform it professionally to gain insight into the client's or patient's perspective. It can enable students to begin to consider the attitudes and feelings that surface on such occasions and to enable them to analyze and practise the social skills necessary in the professional situation. Despite these advantages, this technique does not appear to be used as frequently as it might, which may be because acting and playing may be considered to be childish or only adult if they occur in the right place, like a theatre. Additionally, it may also not be used because it appears artificial and the actors feel inhibited or because it is recognized that such dramatic interaction might provoke an emotional situation that the teachers do not feel confident enough to handle.

To some extent the sense of artificiality can be overcome in the work of preceptors and teacher practitioners if they explain to the students that role play is a teaching and learning method that provides a safe situation for them to work out their role performance in a new situation, to enact a difficult situation, and to aid reflection upon a previously problematic experience. During the initial preparation for the role play the teacher practitioners should explain the rationale behind the session and give precise details of the ideas and roles that they and the students are going to perform. They should also indicate that participants are free to stop the role play at any time, but whenever they complete it there will be a period afterwards during which they can discuss quietly the situation that has been enacted, the process through which they have gone and the emotions that they have experienced. Debriefing, according to Van Ments (1989) is the most important part of the process for it is during this period that reflective learning occurs. Van Ments suggests that there are three phases in debriefing: asking, analyzing and concluding. First all the actors (protagonists and observers) have to be asked what happened and agree upon it. Secondly, the process is analyzed and, if necessary, re-run. Finally, conclusions are drawn and recommendations made.

Like all effective teaching techniques, this one demands very careful planning by the teacher practitioners and preceptors, the more so in this instance because the emotions and attitudes of individuals may be displayed in a more open manner than is considered natural and normal in contemporary society. The usefulness of the approach may be seen in the way that it incorporates actual professional situations into the teaching and learning situation. Many examples could be given but two only will be provided here. Consider the distressing situation of a health visitor going to a young mother who had, on the previous evening, found her three-month-old son dead in his cot; the student could play the health visitor and the teacher practitioner play the mother. Another situation might be that of the district nurse visiting a patient who has carcinoma of the lung and who suspects his condition, although he has never been informed of it by his doctor. The patient asks the district nurse if he has cancer: the student might play the role of the district nurse and the teacher practitioner that of the patient. These examples are possible situations in professional practice and they are provided only to illustrate the use of this technique in the preparation of professionals. In some role play it might be useful for students to play the role of the patient in order to gain empathy and to understand more about their own professional role.

Some teacher practitioners or preceptors may not feel confident in the use of role play technique and they may, therefore, seek to avoid using it. However, it has considerable use in professional training, so it is a technique with which they should be familiar, and which they should consider employing. However, it should be used with caution because it can create emotional release, so it might be wise for the teachers to participate in role playing exercises before they introduce it into their own teaching.

Whilst role play is often more spontaneous than simulation, the latter can also be valuable in learning and teaching. It is, however, more time-consuming to prepare, although once ready it can be used on numerous occasions with successive groups of students – provided that it is updated when necessary. One example might be that of a newly qualified social worker arriving at her office to find that her colleagues in her team had been taken ill in the night and she had to fulfil their commitments. Having access to their diaries she has to decide how to prioritize her time for that day. Once the diaries were prepared, it would be possible to simulate this exercise with different groups of students.

CASE STUDIES

Case studies are based upon examination and analysis of a real or a simulated problem. There are a number of different approaches that can be used in a one-to-one teaching and learning situation. These cases can be designed and used with different groups of students. For example, a social worker receives a letter of complaint and she is expected to deal with it. Another might be that a health visitor has to prioritize the contents of her in-tray after returning from a two-week holiday. Naturally, students in practice situations are also likely to prepare case studies of specific clients or patients, or even of practices and jobs. In all of these situations, teacher practitioners and mentors can play significant roles.

STUDENT ASSIGNMENTS

The practical assignment is one in which the teachers encourage the students to undertake a piece of work on their own; it may be written, research-orientated or skill-based and it may be teacher-directed or student-initiated. In some training courses where it is considered that the theory is taught by one teacher and the practice is taught by someone in the clinical work situation, there is a tendency for the latter not to be expected to be involved in setting assignments or work for the student. However, motivating students to undertake an assignment is a method of facilitating students' learning and should be encouraged so long as students are given sufficient time to undertake the task and it does not interfere with the assessment procedure of the course which has been approved by the award-granting and statutory bodies. Such an activity may arise from: a controlled discussion session; from articles; from suggestions by the teacher practitioners or preceptors that the students should find out about a specific procedure or practice; from a much more didactic talk after which the teachers suggest that the students should read a number of articles on a specific topic and make a synopsis of them; from a demonstration of skill, after which students are asked to practise it until it has been mastered, etc. However, it is also possible for assignments to precede a teaching session where, for instance, the teacher practitioners might explain to students that in a few days time they will be given a specific role or responsibility and that they should discover what is entailed; the teacher practitioners might then plan a socratic guided discussion a few days later in anticipation that the students would have already acquired some knowledge about it. Thus it may be seen that not all assignments have to be assessed coursework, but that a variety of assignments may be used, often in conjunction with other teaching methods, by the teacher practitioners.

VISITS AND TRIPS

Teacher practitioners may also be facilitators of the students' learning by providing opportunity for the latter to have a learning need met outside of the actual professional practice situation in which they perform. This may be undertaken on the basis that they understand the students' learning needs and are aware of other people who, or situations which, might be able to help the students satisfy that specific need effectively. They may, for instance, arrange for a student to visit a centre of excellence, an expert in a discipline or skill, a colleague who has within her or his professional practice and care patients whose physical or social condition is such that the students should have knowledge and expertise. Finally, the teacher practitioners or preceptors may arrange for the students to visit each other so that they can exchange information and ideas.

When visits and trips are arranged, it is necessary for the teacher practitioners or preceptors to make careful arrangements, using the appropriate official channels in order to ensure that the relevant personnel are aware of what has been arranged and the purpose of the students' visit. The teacher practitioners and preceptors should also prepare the students prior to the visit, so that they are enabled to obtain maximum benefit from the experience. Additionally, the teacher practitioners should ensure that after such a visit they conduct a follow-up session in order to assist the students to reflect on what they experienced and crystalize their ideas from the learning experience that has been provided. Finally, the teacher practitioners must ensure that the normal after-visit courtesies are undertaken by both themselves and the students, so that the person who received the visitors is aware of its usefulness and that it has been appreciated.

It may be seen from the above discussions that a combination of teaching methods may be more useful than employing only one technique per topic. A variety of approaches may enrich the learning experience, so that the more proficient the teacher practitioners and preceptors are in utilizing different techniques the more efficiently will the students be prepared to perform their professional role. Since teacher practitioners may be facilitators of the students' learning rather than merely providers of information and instructors of skills for the students to learn, they may not only enable the students to learn all that they know, but they may also actually teach the students more than they know, and that can only be enriching for the profession as a whole and for the patients and clients whom the students will serve when they are qualified.

SOME OTHER TEACHING METHODS

Teacher practitioners and preceptors are sometimes invited to give a presentation before a group of people, for example, students in a college or a school of nursing, clients in a health centre, so they should be aware of some of the techniques of teaching groups, but since this is not their main teaching role less emphasis is placed upon it here. Even so, some reference is made to some of the main approaches that they may wish to employ, although if they are particularly interested in this they might be wise to read some of the texts recommended in the selection of further reading at the end of this book. The two main methods mentioned here, the lecture and lecture-discussion, have a number of variations although the same dichotomy of teacher-centred and learner-centred approaches is appropriate.

THE LECTURE

This is the normal approach expected from visiting speakers since they have some knowledge and information that they are expected to convey to the learners within a specified time. However, there are a number of variations on the lecture, including: the normal straight lecture, the lecture followed by discussion and the lecture interspersed with discussion. Each of these are now examined briefly.

The normal lecture technique is perhaps the most common form of teaching and yet, despite its popularity, many criticisms have been levelled at it, so it is important to put this method into perspective. Bligh (1971 p4), who considers that lecturing is an art and that the skill is acquired through practice rather than books, summarizes research on the topic when he argues that:

- with the exception of programmed learning the lecture is as effective as any other method of transmitting information, but not more effective
- most lectures are not as effective as more active methods for the production of thought
- changing student attitudes should not normally be the major objective of the lecture.

Thus it may be seen that only in the transmission of information is the lecture as effective as other methods of teaching, but it must also be recognized that much of the research that led to this conclusion was not actually conducted with adult students. However, Trenaman's research (see above) on the length of time that people will listen to a talk was, in fact, with adults (see Legge, 1974).

Lecturing has had some bad press in recent years, but it is always worth recalling what Powell wrote about it:

As with kissing, clinical tests can prove that lecturing is 'bad thing'. Indeed, the comparison can be taken further. Those who have never participated in a good lecture cannot know its power to inspire: its full impact can only be appreciated by consenting adults; its effectiveness is usually dependent upon effective visual aids ... (Cited from Mills, 1977 p156)

Indeed, Costin (1972 p25) concluded that studies for 40 years have supported Spence's claim that decrying the use of lectures was not justified, but decrying their wholesale use was. Consequently, the positive use of lecturing should be acknowledged.

If teacher practitioners or preceptors are invited to give a lecture, they may feel duty-bound to concur with the request and use the traditional approach, since this will almost certainly be what the audience expect from them. If they deliver a lecture, there are a number of points relevant to the preparation discussed in the earlier section on the talk. In addition a number of common errors that should be avoided are listed below:

- *Preparing too much material*: Conscientious lecturers may prepare far too much material for the time that they have been allocated and, as they are making their presentation, they might realize that they have insufficient time to deliver it all. Consequently they try to speed up the pace of the lecture and, by so doing, they lose the learners' concentration. If teacher practitioners find themselves in this position, it is better to try to slow down and summarize the main points.
- *Speaking for too long*: As Trenaman showed, concentration spans vary from about five to about 20 minutes, so there tends to be a lessening of concentration after the first few minutes and this may result in much of the material presented being lost to the audience. A brief pause, a change of teaching and learning method, a joke or a stop for questions will all help retain interest.
- *Being bound to notes*: Teacher practitioners should try to avoid being bound to notes to prevent them losing eye contact with their listeners and, therefore, being less sensitive to their expressed needs. If the volume of notes is reduced, then there is more likely to be a genuine interchange between speaker and learners.
- *Speaking with one's back to the audience*: This occurs most frequently if speakers use a whiteboard or chalkboard, and it often results in adults, especially those with slightly impaired hearing, losing some of the words uttered by the speakers. If the lecturers want to use a board, it is worth remaining silent whilst writing, although an alternative approach would be to employ an overhead projector.
- *Walking around the room while speaking*: This may also result in students, especially those who are hard of hearing, finding it difficult to follow every word that the lecturers speak. Even so, this is not to suggest the lecturers should remain immobile during the delivery, only that the teachers are aware of the potential problem. Some teachers, however, do prefer to remain seated all the time.
- *Not speaking loudly enough*: This is a common occurrence with inexperienced lecturers and it may be useful for the teachers to pick out a member of the audience who is rather close to the back of the

room and imagine that they are addressing that one individual, although they should not focus solely upon that person, since this might cause embarrassment.

- *Speaking too quickly*: Often speakers try to ensure everybody hears by merely trying to speak more loudly, but it is also most beneficial for them to slow down the speed of their presentation and to ensure that the ends of the words are clearly pronounced.

Whilst lectures have a number of limitations, some of which may be partially overcome by variations upon the technique, the fact that it is a teacher-centred approach must also be recognized.

The lecture-discussion is an approach quite frequently expected of visiting lecturers, although the concluding discussion often tends to take the form of questions being raised by members of the audience and addressed to the speakers, usually seeking clarification and amplification of a point raised in the presentation itself. However, this technique may take the form of a short presentation by speakers followed by group discussion with, or without, a concluding plenary session. If the teacher practitioners wish to employ this approach they should ensure that the institution inviting them is prepared for the use of the methods, that the room is suitable and that the chairs are not fixed together. This is a problem in those rooms where chairs are fixed in order to meet fire regulations. If this technique is used, teacher practitioners should prepare carefully the question(s) that the groups are to discuss and ensure that they are directly related to some issue(s) raised in the initial address. Where small groups are used in this way, the teachers should ensure that all the group members know each other and if they do not, they should be encouraged to introduce themselves to each other at the outset. If there is to be a plenary session during which the conclusions of each group are to be reported, the teacher practitioners should ensure that a rapporteur is elected from each group, and, if necessary, that there is a group secretary and chairperson. However, if the time is limited they may wish to delegate these roles in a more arbitrary manner.

When presentation and discussion are interspersed, it is much harder for lecturers to form small groups and move chairs, etc., so the teacher practitioners and preceptors might wish to ask questions and pose problems to the listeners at pre-selected times during the address. This is a useful approach and it does help overcome the problem of lapsed concentration. However, if the room in which the lecture is given is arranged with chairs in rows lecturers are unlikely to generate much group discussion because there is little or no eye contact between the listeners, so that all the response will be directed to speakers. If, on the other hand, the chairs are so arranged to allow participants to see each other, then the teacher practitioners may manage to get interaction between the group as a result of the questions. This may be less likely with a large audience and in this instance responses to the questions may be dominated by the less retiring members of the audience. This approach does allow the lecturers to plan their time carefully, even though they may be forced to intervene in a discussion in order to pursue the goals of the session, if they are still considered to be important. However, if there is good and valid discussion it may be perfectly legitimate not to follow a preconceived plan.

DISCUSSION METHODS

It will already have been recognized how important discussion methods are to the teaching of adults. There are two other approaches that are referred to here even though they have similarities to the above techniques. Bligh (1971 p126) mentions the use of *free-group discussion*, which he defines as a learning situation in which the topic and the direction are controlled by the student group. While this is a useful method for teachers, it is not necessarily one that the teacher practitioners are likely to employ when they are invited to speak at a local college or department of nursing. By contrast, they might well utilize a problem-centred discussion technique, where they set groups problems to solve prior to them entering the discussion with the students. This approach does encourage analytical thinking, ability to make decisions, and the opportunity to evaluate them. It is a useful method for teacher practitioners to employ in a situation where they are able to have a longer time with the learners.

Brainstorming is another useful, albeit intensive, discussion technique in which spontaneous suggestions or solutions to problems are discussed and recorded. This is a well-known method in professional groups, since it is designed to produce lateral thinking and innovative perspectives upon problems and issues.

Having examined a number of different teaching methods that teacher practitioners might find useful in the course of their work, it is now necessary to consider the use of teaching aids.

TEACHING AIDS

Teaching aids are used most frequently in a more formal classroom setting, but they are also useful in non-formal teaching and learning. The purpose of this section is to examine briefly some of the aids that might be useful to teacher practitioners, but not to refer to the wider variety of audio-visual aids that may be employed in the classroom. Four groups of aids are discussed here: audio-cassettes, charts, handouts and models.

AUDIO CASSETTES

At present there are few audio cassettes available for purchase that would be useful for the work of the teacher practitioners. Nevertheless, this does not prevent them preparing their own and this would be especially useful for teacher practitioners whose work is located in the community and who are, therefore, expected to use a car. In many instances, students also have their own cars and thus, it is quite possible for the teacher practitioners to prepare their own cassettes and to loan them to students when the students are working independently. Subjects that might be covered, include: helping prepare the students for a difficult visit; helping the students assess the visit by raising a series of questions which they should consider in assessing their practice; a socratic-type exercise to follow a teaching and learning session in which they have both been engaged; an exercise to consider an article in a journal in a critical manner, etc. Once prepared, the use of the audio cassette is both time saving and an approach that helps the students create a habit of independent learning. This method may also be useful in a health centre or a hospital setting where preceptors and teacher practitioners could prepare a number of cassettes about specific relevant aspects of practice which the students could use when an appropriate time arose, for example, describing a specific procedure or raising questions about it. (The student should be advised to ensure that audio cassette recorders and tapes are kept in a safe place and that, where relevant, confidentiality is assured.)

Both in the community and hospital settings, the use of this technique depends upon the availability of resources and the willingness of teacher practitioners to employ less common approaches to teaching. It might also be possible for teacher practitioners to use the expertise of audio-visual staff in universities, colleges and health education units to help in the preparation of such cassettes. It might be possible for a teaching centre to build a library of such aids.

CHARTS AND DIAGRAMS

Some people learn better through visual perception than they do by listening, so it is useful for teacher practitioners to prepare or collect their own library of charts and diagrams. These may refer to any aspect of theory or practice. While a local university or college department of nursing, or social and community work, may have its own resource centre which the teachers can use, they may discover that they need visual aids that relate specifically to the type of work which they are undertaking and those with a directly practical orientation, so that it may be better if they obtained or prepared and stored them for themselves. Not all visual aids have to be made by the teacher practitioners; many charts and diagrams are produced by commercial companies, especially in order to advertise their own products. These are often supplied freely, or may be obtained inexpensively, so it is useful for teachers to be aware of these sources of visual information and to collect as much relevant material as possible. These are often mentioned in the professional press and may be purchased from local and national organizations. Having collected a library of charts and diagrams, it is necessary to have a storage facility, such as a cupboard or a filing cabinet, which is readily available to the teacher practitioners. But once material is stored there are a number of points that should be borne in mind when they use the material on a later occasion, including whether it is:

- still accurate and up-to-date
- completely relevant to the individualized teaching and learning situation for which it is intended
- appropriate to make the points that the teacher practitioners wish it to make in the specific situation.

HANDOUTS

The handout is a useful teaching aid, since many students find that they learn best by reading about the subject and reflecting upon it, either before or after a teaching session, so teacher practitioners may wish to give students a handout prior to a session with an agreement to discuss it on a specific forthcoming occasion, or they may provide a handout after a session for students to study. Most handouts have to be prepared by the teacher practitioners and initially this may be a time-consuming process, but once a handout has been prepared and copies of it made, it can be used on subsequent occasions. Handouts can be word-processed, or handwritten, but they should be neatly prepared. Obviously, with many computer programs available, wordprocessed handouts are becoming more professional. Photographs and diagrams can be included in a handout, if appropriate, provided that they can be printed or photocopied. However, it has to be recognized that there are increasing financial constraints on the use of such materials and students might be given the option of purchasing handouts or returning them after they have used them.

Another type of a handout that the teacher practitioners may find useful is prepared reading material, such as an article in a journal, a research report or a chapter of a book, or even a list of references. Having directed students to such material or loaned a copy to the student, it is desirable for the teacher practitioners to conduct a socratic-style teaching and learning session about it at a later date in order to ensure that the students have critically understood the material provided.

MODELS

Many departments of nursing and social work have models relevant to many aspects of the course of study in their resource centres, to which students often have ready access. Occasionally, however, teacher practitioners may wish to use models in relation to the work that they are undertaking with a student. If they have access to the resource centre, or relevant museum, then it is useful for them to have borrowing rights for equipment, but if there is no such centre, or they do not have ready access to it, they may wish to construct their own models. This need not be an expensive undertaking since many models can be constructed from materials that might normally be thrown away as useless. Such a task is time-consuming, but it will be rewarding if the end product is enriched learning by the students, as teacher practitioners who have prepared such material have discovered.

It will be noted from a number of references in this section that teacher practitioners may wish to store the material that they collect or prepare. Hence, they may wish to prepare their own small resource centres. Additionally, they should be aware of places where they can acquire teaching aids such as a resource centre and libraries in educational institutions, local Health Education Departments, national resource centres, etc.

PREPARING A TEACHING AND LEARNING SESSION

It will have become clear from the foregoing discussion that in order to ensure that a teaching and learning session has a good chance of success, it is necessary for teacher practitioners and mentors to undertake considerable preparation, so that it is now important to focus upon this process. Basically a number of elements have to be considered and these include: the aims and objectives of the session, content, method, location, timing and evaluation. Each of these points is discussed in turn.

AIMS AND OBJECTIVES

Since the aims of a course usually reflect its broad philosophical intentions, they are of less significance to the teacher practitioners' immediate preparation than are the course objectives. Even so, they should have agreed with the students the aims of the practical professional experience which is being provided. These should reflect the overall aims of the course and since these do not usually vary from one session to the

next, it is the objectives of the teaching session that should be the immediate concern of the teacher practitioners' preparation. Clearly these also
need to be in accord with the previously formulated aims.

It will be recalled that certain reservations were raised about behavioural objectives in Chapter 3, mostly because learning is much wider
than behaviour, so it might be wiser for teacher practitioners to formulate the objectives in non-behavioural terms, unless there is agreement
between them and the students in respect of a specific skill or procedure. In this instance they may wish to agree upon specific behavioural
objectives. Naturally, the teacher practitioners should discuss with the
students the programme of events for two or three days in advance in
order that they might agree upon objectives for specific sessions.
Objectives should have a degree of specificity and be the guidelines for
the teacher practitioners in preparing individual teaching and learning
programmes.

Some departments of nursing and midwifery provide specific objectives for the various designated clinical areas and those responsible for
the teaching and learning in these locations are expected to use these.
Usually they have been developed co-operatively by various grades of
staff. If teacher practitioners or the students are dissatisfied with any of
the objectives with which they are presented, they should discuss these
with the personnel who provided them, so that amendments might be
made to ensure that they are relevant to the situation.

CONTENT

Having prepared the objectives, teacher practitioners may then select
relevant content matter and order it in a logical sequence, so that it
starts from the point at which the previous session had concluded, or
from a point about which teacher practitioners know the students are
already knowledgeable, or from a relevant situation. The progression of
the content should be carefully prepared even though the sequence may
not be retained during the teaching and learning session because of
interventions from the student. Many teachers feel more confident, especially early in their careers, if they have prepared and produced detailed
notes prior to a teaching session. This is a form of preparation to be
recommended, even though in the non-formal teaching and learning
situation full notes may not actually be employed, since each situation
actually provides a new learning situation for the teacher. When teacher
practitioners are not perfectly sure of the content themselves they should
consult a relevant authority (literature or person) prior to teaching so
that they do not knowingly provide the student with incorrect information. Being certain that they have the correct information is also a
confidence boosting phenomenon for teachers and mentors.

METHODS

At the same time as the teachers are selecting the content, they should also be planning the method(s) that they are going to employ and these should be built into the lesson plan. Consideration should be given to a number of factors when selecting the method, including:

- the student's preferred learning style
- the approaches the teacher practitioners would prefer to employ
- the way that the selected content might best be presented in order to achieve the desired objectives
- which teaching aids would enhance the teaching and learning session
- the location which is available for the session.

LOCATION AND TIMING

If teacher practitioners have a choice of locations for the teaching and learning session, then deciding upon which location to use is an important element in its preparation. It is also important to recognize that in planning the location, consideration will also need to be given to the seating arrangements to ensure eye contact, whether the session should take place over a cup of coffee, etc. The session should also be kept to the planned length so it does not interfere with any of the other professional commitments of any participant.

EVALUATION

After any teaching and learning process the teacher practitioners and preceptors should evaluate what has been undertaken. Evaluation is not merely asking whether the objectives of the session have been achieved but whether all aspects of the teaching and learning session had been satisfactory. Evaluation is something of a research process, obtaining information which can be useful in deciding future plans relating to the sessions being evaluated. Included in the questions that the teacher practitioners should ask are:

- Did the objectives reflect the overall aims of the course?
- Were the objectives achieved?
- Were the objectives satisfactory?
- Was the content sufficient?
- Was the content relevant?
- Was the presentation of the content structured in a logical manner?
- Were the methods employed the most effective?
- Which other approaches might have been utilized effectively?
- What effect has the session had upon the learners' knowledge or practice?

- Was the time and/or place of the session appropriate?
- Was the relationship between participants conducive to effective learning?
- How else might the whole situation have been improved?
- How else might the teaching and learning session have been improved?

At the end of such an evaluation, teacher practitioners should be in a position to determine the strengths and the weaknesses of the teaching and learning session that they have conducted. Evaluation is a matter of knowing both the strengths and the weaknesses of a session. It is as important for the teacher practitioners to be as aware of their strengths as of their weaknesses, so that they can continue to improve their own performance.

Occasionally, such an evaluation session might be conducted jointly by teacher practitioners and students so that the former has another perception of the performance. The extent to which the students should be involved will depend upon the relationship between the two, but it would be quite out of keeping with the ideals of professional education if it were not to occur.

There is a real sense in which evaluation should be part of the quality assurance process, something which higher education is placing great great emphasis upon at the current time. The Universities Association of Continuing Education (de Wit, 1993 p27) stresses the importance of evaluating the total learning experience, so that the teacher practitioners' and preceptors' role should be give high priority.

Conclusion

This chapter has examined the teaching role of teacher practitioners, a role that is significant to the preparation of new recruits to a profession. However, the majority of teacher practitioners also perform another significant role during this period of preparation, that of assessor; Chapter 6 explores the nature of assessment.

Assessing students 6

This chapter explores:
- *The nature of assessment*
- *Rationale for assessment*
- *Assessment of prior learning and prior experiential learning*
- *Types of assessment*
- *Techniques in assessment*
- *Peer and self-assessment*
- *Teaching the art of self-assessment.*

INTRODUCTION

Not only do teacher practitioners and preceptors teach students, they are frequently required to act as assessors, which in some instances entails reporting on the students' suitability for admission to the profession. The responsibility for making such a judgment is one that should not be assumed lightly by anybody, so it is an aspect of the role that some do not like to perform. This reluctance is perfectly understandable since the teacher practitioners' or preceptors' report may, in some circumstances adversely affect a students' career and even prevent individuals actually entering the profession. Nevertheless, its performance is an element of the same responsibility that they have to the patients/clients, that of ensuring that they are always rendered the best possible service.

THE NATURE OF ASSESSMENT

Many people in education have tried to equate assessment with some forms of measurement, but in this section it is argued that this is a false perspective to adopt and what teacher practitioners and preceptors do really is to place a value upon different phenomena. Naturally the phenomena (for example, levels of skill demonstrated in performing a procedure) differ, but this is only really recognized through seeing a lot of different people perform the same practice, or by having a standard which qualified practitioners are expected to achieve. In order to try to demonstrate the nature of assessment, a comparison is made here with the art of measuring.

Most children learn how to use a protractor at school in order to measure or draw angles. They know that when they measure an angle for a second time, they should get the same result as they did the first, since the same angle is fixed and unchanging. If they want to be more accurate in their measurement, they use a more sophisticated instrument. In the same manner if they want to measure length accurately and precisely, they can use a micrometer. A variety of micrometers, gauges and callipers, and even more accurate instruments, exist to allow the scientist to measure an external object with degrees of the utmost precision. Doctors and nurses also engage in this activity when they measure a precise dose of a drug to be administered to a patient. The phenomenon that they measure, in these cases, is empirical and the measurements that they take can be replicated to ensure that they are correct. The measurement is of an objective phenomenon and is apparently objective knowledge, but more precisely, it is subjective knowledge about an objective phenomenon. In exactly the same way, chemists can take any substance and analyze its contents and specify precisely its constitution. Once again, providing that the analysis is correct, the outcome will always be the same, since the substance is objective and unchanging – but the knowledge is still subjective.

Measurement is always the same and this can be read from an instrument, learned, or memorized, without being altered by the differences of perception, the latter being a human characteristic. It is as if the knowledge were external, although it is subjective knowledge about the same external unchanging phenomena.

If teachers seek to assess students' academic work, such as an essay, it would look rather strange if the assessment read rather like this: the essay is 5,231 words long, has been printed in courier typeface on 17 pages and eight lines. But it is accurate, replicable and unchanging. It is an accurate measurement of an objective phenomenon, but it tells us little about the content or the standard – whatever that is! In a similar manner, it would look strange if teacher practitioners tried to measure skill performance in this way. Assessment cannot be equated with measurement, regardless of the sophistication of the instruments produced to give an appearance of measuring performance.

Assessment is a normal part of any social interaction. Whenever a person is introduced to another individual and thereafter spends some time in social intercourse with that individual, there is likely to occur a reflective comment on either the nature of the person or of the social interaction, for example, 'he was a nice fellow', 'she is really quite remarkable', or 'that conversation was enjoyable'. These comments are the essence of assessment: that they are assessing a person, an inter-action or a situation. Assessors place a value upon something that did not necessarily have one for them before. In the case of the examples given here, the value is that which one person places upon another, i.e. nice or remarkable. Other people may, or may not, agree with the assess-ment since it is quite subjective.

It will be noted that assessment and evaluation are similar processes – indeed, they are! However, it is conventional in education to restrict evaluation to teaching and learning sessions, courses and programmes, and to use assessment in respect of assignments, projects, work perfor-mance, etc. This is quite a crude distinction, but educational literature usually conforms to this convention.

Yet assessments of students should not be quite as subjective as the above examples suggest, or else entry to the profession would be rather a precarious business. However, in other branches of education and in other forms of examination, such as the written essay-type examination, it is recognized that subjectivity plays a significant part in assessment. Even very experienced examiners can differ by a considerable amount when marking the same essay (see, for example, Jarvis, 1978), so that even written examinations have been designed using other techniques in order to make them more objective, for example, multiple-choice ques-tions. However, whilst some approaches may be useful, they are not without their problems. Additionally, Dobby (1981 p6) discovered that trainee district nurses were rated by their practical work teacher more highly than did a group of visiting practical work teachers. Practical work teachers were also more likely to rate good trainees higher and poor trainees poorer at everything. Since subjectivity is recognized as being part of the assessment process, it should not cause teacher prac-titioners undue stress, unless it is directed towards or against people rather than their practice, a point that will be discussed later in this chapter. In practical work assessments many attempts have been made to ensure that there is some objectivity and many departments of nursing and social work have issued checklists of competencies (skills/procedures) that should be taught and assessed during practice. However, Dobby (1981 p5) noted considerable variation in the number of competences being assessed by the district nurse training centres. This problem is likely to have increased with the move to internal valida-tion. These lists may provide useful guidelines, but they do not eradicate the element of subjectivity because the teacher practitioners must still be satisfied with the way in which the students perform the requisite skill/procedure and also their approach to the overall well-being of patient or client. If a grade is awarded as a result of this subjective assessment, it gives the appearance of objective measurement – but this is a process of objectification rather than objectivity!

The grade is related to teacher practitioners' own expectations of how that skill, etc., should be performed. This should be the case whether, or not, they are working to a checklist, undertaking a ward-based assessment, working in a continuous assessment situation or working with the students in a normal professional practice situation. Thus the standards that the teacher practitioners utilize in the assessment of students are almost certainly related in some way to those exhibited in their own professional practice and these should be the rigorous standards of the highly professional practitioner. Dobby (1981 p9) actually proposed a peripatetic moderating system – but even this supposes that any individual is always consistent, which is to be doubted.

It might well be asked whether all assessment is subjective in this manner and the response must clearly depend upon the nature of the knowledge, skill or attitude being assessed. Certain forms of knowledge are indisputable, for example, the specifications of a law or the administration of precise dosages of a certain drug, so that the students are either correct or incorrect when stating these. In these instances teacher practitioners are able to specify quite objectively that the students either do or do not know specific legislation or the administration of certain precise drug dosages. Here there is no requirement of personal perception, it is rather like measuring since it is recording an objective phenomenon. But in many other instances no such possibilities exist, since there may, for instance, be a variety of ways of undertaking a task or implementing a procedure and a multitude of different approaches to a patient/client. In these cases, teacher practitioners may wish to attempt to be objective by stating that the student implemented a procedure in a specific manner or interacted with a patient/client in a certain way and that in the outcome the procedure was completed or that the interaction resulted in specific information being transmitted to the patient/client. Rowntree (1977 p6) calls this descriptive assessment. But the teacher practitioners are still recording their own perception of the event and they are also expected to make a judgment on the practice or interaction, and it is at this point that the subjectivity enters. They may wish to specify that the student implemented the procedure in a manner other than that which they themselves would employ, but that the implementation and its outcome were efficient and satisfactory. Here the assessment is a combination of the descriptive and the judgmental, and it is in the latter that teacher practitioners' own standards are important. While this gives an appearance of objectivity, there is still a personal element within it for the assessors are recording their perceptions of the event.

Indeed, teachers might be affected by other students whom they have also assessed and so their assessments might be influenced by those experiences. The tendency to compare different practices underlies what is known as *norm-based assessment*. In contrast to this is *criterion-based assessment*. In the latter, which is the one that teacher practitioners will probably use most frequently, a number of criteria are specified and provided the students achieve them then they are credited with having achieved the criteria for that specific level of performance. However, this is no less subjective because it still involves the teacher practitioner passing judgment in respect to the standard of the level of performance achieved.

Norm-based assessment is a technique where a number of pieces of work are rank-ordered and then the grades are worked out against the spectrum of the whole group. This is a technique that some external examiners use in order to evaluate the consistency of a course team's marking. The difference between the two can be shown in the following example: a student says that she got a grade of 85 per cent and this appears to be a good mark – against the specified criteria. However, when she then points out that everybody else got over 90 per cent and that she was bottom, she does not appear to have done quite so well!

It will be noted immediately that these various forms of assessment, like some forms of teaching, are teacher-centred, but later in this chapter reference will be made to some learner-centred methods of assessment. Before this is undertaken, however, it is necessary to explore the rationale for assessment.

RATIONALE FOR ASSESSMENT

Earlier in the book it was argued that at the heart of the teaching and learning process there is a diagnostic function, in which teachers and learners actually assess together the strengths and weaknesses of the latter in order to plan future learning experiences. This diagnostic appraisal, which may also be called *formative assessment*, is self-evidently fundamental to individualized teaching and learning. It is something that does not only occur at the outset of students' professional practical experience but should be a continuing process throughout the whole period, so that the learning experiences provided for the students may be most relevant for them. By undertaking this activity the teacher practitioners and preceptors and the students gain feedback about the latter's learning and about their future learning needs, whereas the former also gain similar information and are also able to assess the efficiency of their own teaching methods, etc. In addition to providing feedback to both participants, it should also help to motivate the students to continue to learn in order to satisfy both themselves and the teacher practitioners of their ability. These three factors are teaching- and learning-orientated, and in the first instance they are the most significant reasons for undertaking such a process, even though they may not be the most commonly assumed reasons why assessment is necessary.

Inevitably the teaching and occupational competences of teacher practitioners vary considerably. Therefore, teachers and students should be encouraged to identify the former's strengths and weaknesses, so that the expertise of the teachers can be sought when it is appropriate.

Perhaps the most common reason given for assessment is that of the maintenance of standards. Obviously any profession must ensure that new recruits to its ranks have, prior to entry, achieved professionally accepted standards. This is the prime responsibility that the profession has to its clients/patients in order to provide the best service and, thereby, maintain public trust and support. While it is common practice for institutions of higher education to assume responsibility for admitting new learners to the profession based upon the outcomes of all aspects of the qualifying examinations, the professional associations or the statutory bodies still retain the responsibility for accrediting these institutions. Having been accredited, much of the responsibility of both preparing the students in the professional practice situation and assessing them in it rests with teacher practitioners and preceptors. It is they who, as a result of their own experience and education, may recommend that specific learners should be accepted into the profession, either because they have achieved standards acceptable to themselves as experienced professionals who have been given that responsibility by the profession, or because learners are improving and should achieve those standards before they enter the practice. In this latter instance it is important that teacher practitioners should expect high standards from their students and that in order to achieve them they should maintain high standards themselves. To expect high standards is important since it ensures that those whom the teacher practitioners recommend for entry to the profession have achieved, or are in the process of achieving, a level of competency in practice that should stand them in good stead when they become fully fledged members of the profession.

At the same time it has to be remembered that there is little evidence to show that standards achieved in initial preparation will necessarily relate to standards achieved in practice thereafter, since professional opportunities for continuing education in the context of the practice, etc. means that people's standards of practice can change for better or for worse, and also be changed, by events beyond initial training. Consequently, it is as important to help learners gain positive attitudes to their work and help them learn to learn, so that they can continue to develop in their practice.

ASSESSMENT OF PRIOR LEARNING AND PRIOR EXPERIENTIAL LEARNING

Increasingly courses are being designed utilizing a modular approach and, as a result, institutions are more prepared to give remission of some part of the curriculum based upon previous learning, whether it be from a formal educational setting (Assessment of Prior Learning – APL) or through life experience (Assessment of Prior Experiential Learning – APEL). In order to do this it is necessary to assess the extent to which the applicants have learned from these previous situations or experiences. Applicants are expected to justify their application for remission and there are a variety of ways of so doing – including producing certificates from previous courses, preparing a portfolio of previous experiences and having an interview with one or other members of the course team in order to discuss the relevance of the previous learning and experience, etc.

Remission might be granted for two different types of prior learning: the one more general and the other quite specific. For instance, if remission is granted for specific prior learning, it will almost certainly refer to precisely the same type of course, or activity, having already been completed as the one from which remission is sought. General remission, however, is allowed for previous learning activities which relate in general to the course for which remission is being requested.

Teacher practitioners, as members of course teams, might well be requested to make an assessment on part of a portfolio about the level of expertise necessary to undertake some practical activities. However, most of the final decisions will rest with the agreed protocol of the relevant institution.

TYPES OF ASSESSMENT

It has, perhaps, become quite evident that there are a number of different types of assessment and that three have already been mentioned:

- *formative assessment*: diagnostic, undertaken during the teaching and learning programme
- *summative assessment*: a final assessment that occurs at the end of a course, possibly through an examination
- *continuing or continuous assessment*: an on-going process throughout the course.

In the past, nursing specified four practical clinical assessments which may be regarded as summative, even though these may not have actually occurred at the end of the course, since once an assessment had been completed successfully there was no need for it to be repeated.

In some areas continuous assessment is more popular and, as it is in accordance with the demands of diagnostic appraisal, it obviously has its merits since it might continue to form the basis of the teaching and learning programme. It is also a method that has increased in popularity even though it is not without its drawbacks, such as continued stress and potential interference in the relationship between the teacher practitioner and the learner. Individual summative assessments (for example, oral examinations, ward-based assessments) may be short, sharp and painful when they occur, but for some students continuous assessment may be long, drawn-out and nagging. Hence, not all students view continuous assessment as beneficial. Obviously the degree of stress does depend upon the relationship between the teachers and the learners, since if there is a harmonious relationship between them the latter will be aware of how they are progressing and, provided that the progress is satisfactory, they should be able to enjoy their practice with few fears. However, this may not always be the case with the weaker students who may fear failure. They may be worried about being assessed, in the same way that some fear being appraised. Consequently, it might have a detrimental effect on them since they might be unwilling to ask questions, to discuss problems, etc., because they are afraid that they will reveal their weaknesses to their assessor. In these instances, therefore, the role of assessor may interfere with both the relationship and the teacher practitioners' teaching role because the learners' presentation of themselves is slightly false or over-confident. When this occurs, a great deal of responsibility lies with the teacher practitioners or preceptors to overcome this problem and their own sensitivity and social skills are important if they are to be able to help the student use their time as learners most efficiently.

Teacher practitioners and preceptors are expected to keep records of students' progress and, while this is often time consuming, it is important. As courses are being evaluated for their own quality, and much of this type of evaluation can only be undertaken through the checking of records, it is necessary for teacher practitioners to keep a careful record of the activities that students have undertaken and the standard which is achieved. Teacher practitioners and preceptors should do this regularly, even daily, recording both the type of activity performed by the students and their assessment of it. It is advisable to ensure that the date of each record is also kept so that reports can be written with considerable accuracy. If the educational institutions do not issue record books, it might be advisable for teacher practitioners and preceptors to start their own with each new student.

When continuous assessment is introduced into a long course, for example, social work training, it might not be possible for the learners to have the same teacher practitioners, mentors or preceptors and assessors throughout because of the varied programme of placement, so while the assessment may be continuous in one sense, it is inevitably discontinuous in another. Teacher practitioners and assessors may have differing standards and expect different responses from students, so that various parts of the course might be more difficult than others, etc. Additionally, the records that one teacher practitioner or assessor makes may be passed on to another, so that the second teacher practitioner or assessor may be influenced by the judgments of the first, and a self-fulfilling prophecy created. Dobby (1981 p6) highlighted the outcome of the 'halo effect' in his research when he showed that practical work teachers saw everything about good students as good, and everything about poor students as poor. These are not light problems. However, the main reasons for raising them here are to emphasize the discontinuous nature of continuous assessment, and the problem of being so influenced by a earlier report about the student which might well be influenced by personal bias.

Throughout this text considerable emphasis has been placed upon the students assessing their own strengths and weaknesses and discussing them with their teacher practitioners and preceptors, so it must be recognized that not all assessment is necessarily teacher-centred. There is also student-centred assessment. Two forms of student-centred assessment, peer- and self-assessment, are discussed later in this chapter. Obviously self-assessment is an important element in the type of teaching and learning transaction that has been discussed here in which both teacher practitioners and learners collaborate in the formative assessment procedure. Heron (1981) recognized the significance of this type of assessment, which he called collaborative assessment, and while this is at the heart of the individualized teaching and learning transaction, it would be quite false if something of the same form were not to occur at the summative stage. Ultimately the responsibility at that stage lies with teacher practitioners, but the collaborative enterprise may be more accurate in the long term and it may remove some of the fear of the assessor's role that some weaker students have, so that it would be recommended here that, even in the final summative assessment, the same philosophy should prevail in as far as it is possible. Clearly, teacher practitioners may occasionally have the very unpleasant task of recommending that a student be deferred but, in this case, the earlier collaboration should even make this activity a little easier since the student will be aware of the teacher practitioner's own standards and concerns and also of any self-assessments which might have been made. In these difficult situations, well-documented records are essential in order to support the recommendation, and in cases where the referred student decides to appeal against the decision, in accord with course procedures and regulations.

TECHNIQUES IN ASSESSMENT

It will be clearly recognized by now that since the teacher practitioners' role entails being an assessor as well as a teacher, any discrete division between the two functions would be artificial. In order to teach, teacher practitioners must be assessors and assessment should precede as well as follow teaching. It is important, therefore, that teacher practitioners and preceptors are familiar with the techniques of assessment. Initially, there are a number of basic requisites that they should undertake:

- *Look*: Teacher practitioners should always be most observant when they have a student working with them. Such observation need not be formal nor overt; teacher practitioners should, however, always be aware of the learner's actions and when the time is appropriate they may wish to use the observations as a teaching resource.
- *Listen* to what students say both to teachers and to others who are in their company. Often what they say will convey to teacher practitioners and mentors information about students' learning needs and attitudes.
- *Listen* to what others say about the students. Patients, colleagues and others may all comment to the teacher practitioners. Clearly the patients'/clients' observations are important, not because they necessarily know the technicalities of professional practice but because they are the recipients of the service. Colleagues may also comment and these should also be listened to with great care. However, the morality of asking for comments from other people is questionable, unless it has first been discussed with the students.
- *Discuss* with the students what they have seen or heard. This is part of the diagnostic process that should be a continuous element in the teaching and learning transaction.
- *Decide*: Ultimately a conclusion has to be reached and this should be as a result of discussion. However, if assessors are in doubt, it is always professional to take a second opinion, even though the first assessor may run the risk of appearing uncertain or even not knowing her own mind. Even so, this should not be used as a method of abrogating the teacher practitioners' own responsibility.

Having highlighted the above process, it is also important to examine some of the more specific elements in the assessment procedure. The aspects focused upon here include: the traditional clinical practice/ward-based assessment and the checklist type of approach that is sometimes used in the assessment of competencies. The latter has been used in the assessment of nurses for many years and may be classified as a criterion-referenced scheme.

If the clinical practice form of assessment is formalized, rather like the traditional four ward-based assessments for general nursing used to be, there is the risk of creating an artificial situation and assessors should do everything in their power to ensure that the artificiality is minimized. So, the assessors' behaviour should be no more formal than it is usually; everything in the clinical situation should be as normal as possible and the whole procedure should occur in as natural a setting as it would in normal professional practice. Assessors should ensure that the learners are put at ease beforehand, but they should also be aware that by trying too hard to free the learners of any anxiety they may actually exacerbate the situation. Hence, even the process of putting the students at ease should be carefully performed, and perhaps this is best done in the days and weeks before the actual assessment occurs by ensuring that the technique or the management process is practised to such a high standard that the students are confident of their own ability to undertake the necessary requirements. No learner should be expected to undertake an assessment unless she has the confidence to pass it and herein lies an important role for the teacher practitioners. They should prepare the learner to pass the assessment and expect them to do so. Belbin and Belbin (1972 pp167–8) note that it does not help students to feel that if they fail they can always try again. In addition, they record the technique adopted by the driving instructor with the most successful record of teaching older persons to drive London Transport buses who claimed that he never mentioned failure and he always acted as if he knew that they were going to pass. By contrast, one with a far higher failure rate claimed that he could spot someone who was going to fail very early in the teaching and learning process. So, the teacher practitioner should prepare the student to pass the assessment.

If the assessment process is formalized and the teacher practitioners are also the assessors, it is interesting to note how the expectations that they have as teacher practitioners may influence their opinions as assessors. For instance, if students perform techniques or procedures well in normal clinical practice, but do not do so well during the formal assessment, should they pass? Likewise, should students who perform better during the assessment than they do in normal clinical practice be given the benefit of any doubt that the assessors may have? Clearly, providing a solution to such complex questions is not easy and yet it is a realistic problem, since examinations of all types should be fair, replicable and relevant to professional practice (Jarvis, 1983a pp106–9).

Often teacher practitioners may have a checklist of competencies that they are expected to ensure that the students have gained during their professional practice, which might be used as the basis for diagnosing the students' strengths and weaknesses. This might form the basis upon which they plan the teaching and learning sessions. In this way the list becomes the focus of tutorial sessions between the teacher practitioners and the students. Hence, it can enrich the process of professional preparation, whereas failure to discuss it might result in impoverished teaching and learning and an incomplete survey of the total demands of practice, because of the type of caseload with which the teacher practitioners are working at the time of the student's professional practical experience.

In continuous assessment, the diagnostic process should continue throughout the period of professional practice. It is very important that teacher practitioners maintain a very full record of the process in order to ensure that the whole area of professional practice is covered by one means or another, and so that they can monitor carefully all aspects of the students' progress. It is perhaps most significant that the teacher practitioners should maintain such a record so that at the end of the practice, or whenever else it is required, they are able to write a full report about the students' performance, but even more important is that through monitoring the students' progress in all aspects of professional practice they are not merely able to report on the students, but they are in a position to offer a prognosis on the likelihood of the students' competence in practice. Prognosis is perhaps an unusual concept to employ in relation to assessment, but since one of the major aims of professional education is to prepare the students to enter professional practice, prediction of the likelihood of the students' competence in it during the early stages of professional practice appears to be a logical expectation from assessment.

Continuous assessment is the most likely form of assessment to offer the basis for any form of prognosis. Hence, it is suggested here that since assessment is about diagnosis and prognosis the teacher practitioners must necessarily be involved in both.

PEER AND SELF-ASSESSMENT

It was noted earlier in this chapter that most of the forms of assessment discussed were teacher-centred, but there have been some objections raised to this approach. Heron (1981), for instance, suggested that teacher-centred assessment is authoritarian, but it is maintained here that although the teacher practitioners and preceptors have authority to assess, such authority must lie in their professionalism rather than their delegated authority as a teacher practitioner, so that teacher-centred assessment is important in professional education. Nevertheless, it is also recognized that the teacher practitioners also have authority delegated from the profession to conduct an assessment, and that the two types of authority are different. However, there is a sense in which teacher-centred assessment is incongruous, if the teacher practitioners and the students have practised collaboration throughout the period of that practice. Therefore, it is necessary to focus upon two learner-centred approaches to assessment, peer and self-assessment. The latter is clearly significant in any form of collaborative assessment, but before this is discussed the former is examined.

PEER ASSESSMENT

This is a form of assessment in which peers, in this case learners, assess each other. It is a useful method when it is possible to have at least two students working together, which teacher practitioners are more likely to have in the hospital situation but which may be less likely in the community. Nevertheless, even in the community it is possible for students to visit each other and to work together occasionally. In these instances, one learner may observe another and then discuss with her the points that she observed. Obviously this may be seen both as an extension of formative assessment but also of discussion methods in teaching and learning. A frequent criticism of this approach is that students are not experts and so this is a case of 'the blind leading the blind'. On a more positive note, there is research that suggests that students may be more realistic in their expectations of their peers than they are of their own work (Rowntree 1977 p146). In addition, teacher practitioners may also learn from what students observe and what they miss in their observations. If this technique is employed, it may also be useful for the teacher practitioners to know something about the dynamics of the whole learner group beforehand because some students may also be influenced by their relationships with each other, as well as the performance that they observe.

Peer assessment might not only occur between students but between teacher practitioners themselves. Indeed, there are some interesting peer mentoring schemes, which might also be called collegial learning (see, for example, Yakowicz in Marsick, 1987). In some of these schemes, devised in schools, teachers are given a 'free' period to watch another teacher perform and vice versa. Underlying the idea is a form of reciprocal support, since colleagues are watching each other teach, learning from it and assessing at the same time, and then teaching each other. Naturally systems like this are open to abuse, but it is only when a collegial atmosphere is built up that this form of peer assessment and teaching can take place within the professional context – when colleagues become each others' mentors.

SELF-ASSESSMENT

Self-assessment encourages students to undertake an appraisal of their own work and then, perhaps, to discuss their assessment with the teacher practitioners or preceptors. Frequently, self-assessment is employed in programmed learning techniques in education where the objectives have been clearly set and the students can assess their own progress. However, it has been consistently maintained in this text that in professional practice the collaborative enterprise between teacher practitioners and learners depends upon there being a continuing process of self-assessment by the students. Rowntree (1977 p146) reports that when students are asked to self-assess and grade written work, there is evidence that some students try to guess the grade that the tutor would have assigned while others are over-generous. Clearly teacher practitioners may find learners who attempt initially to say what they think that the teacher practitioners wants them to say about their practice but, in this instance, it is the responsibility of the teacher practitioners to probe more deeply and to discover what the learners really think. After a period of working together, a more open relationship should be created in which the problem does not arise. Over-generous self-rating of a performance, however, is useful in diagnostic appraisal since it enables the teacher practitioners to become aware of the standards, knowledge and expectations of the students. Thus teacher practitioners are in a position to discuss these with the students, where appropriate.

However, this suggests that self-assessment is only used in a teacher-based manner and this would be a false idea. By listening to the students, teacher practitioners should learn a great deal about what they consider their own needs to be. Since adult students learn best when they see the relevance of what they are doing, it is important that the teacher practitioners respond to the expressed learning needs of the students. Self-assessment is, therefore, quite crucial to the whole process of teaching and learning in an individualized, non-formal manner. Hence the teacher practitioners should, from the outset, encourage this approach; be prepared to listen to what the students say, adopt a socratic approach to assessment after a role performance and continually encourage the students to reflect upon what they have done in order to facilitate their learning process. However, it is suggested here that self-assessment during the professional practice experience should not be isolated from professional practice after qualification, so the teacher practitioners have a further role to play in this respect, but before that is discussed it is necessary to look at self-assessment in a slightly different manner.

Self-assessment also occurs when students evaluate the effect that a learning experience has had on them, as well as when they assess their own knowledge, skills and attitudes. This is a different form of self-assessment and it is as likely to occur in continuing education, when practitioners are released for a course and then return to professional practice. They might then try to assess the effect of the learning experience on them and their practice. This is a transitory process and there are records of instances where two people report on the same course – one two weeks after the event and the other, a social work trainer, two years after. The latter had spent more time reflecting on it and assessing the effects it had had on her and she still recognized that she had not worked it all out. It might be useful, therefore, for teacher practitioners and mentors to recognize that there is a longer term process of self-assessment and they might, consequently, encourage students to reflect on their experiences and see how their attitudes towards previous experiences change as they learn more from their practice.

TEACHING THE ART OF SELF-ASSESSMENT

Professional practitioners endeavour to be the experts (Benner, 1984) in their own field of practice so that they can render the best possible service to their clients. However, the professionals' practice is ultimately the basis upon which their clients and maybe their colleagues will judge them. In order to provide that excellent service they have not only to be good practitioners, but also good theoreticians. Hence, their practice, the implementation of procedures/skills and the way that they interact with clients and colleagues, is fundamental to their professionalism. Therefore professionals need constantly to be able to assess themselves because, once they are fully fledged professionals, they are unlikely to be assessed very frequently by others in such a manner as to benefit their own practice, unless they are lucky enough to have a mentor who is willing to help them or unless they are in the type of collegial situation described earlier in this chapter.

It is, therefore, maintained here that the art of self-assessment should be taught to all intending professional practitioners during their preparation, and for social and community workers, nurses, midwives and health visitors this is one of the tasks of teacher practitioners. Not only do they encourage the students to self-assess their own learning needs but they must help the students assess their practice, so they will develop the habit of reflective practice. This habit will not be developed if teacher practitioners make their comments on the students' role performance before listening to them. Moreover, teacher practitioners, through shrewd questioning, might actually help the students gain more insight into their own practice. In the first instance, teacher practitioners may help students undertake this when they have been present and witnessed the role performance, but as the period of professional experience proceeds they might well wish to help the students assess the practice without actually being present at the role performance. A number of techniques are useful in this instance:

- a socratic tutorial, in which teacher practitioners ask the students about the role performance and continue to raise questions in order to assess it
- a prepared checklist of questions, so that the students are expected to work through the questions after a role performance in order to get into the habit of analyzing the process
- a written record and assessment of each role performance for the teacher practitioners to read. In this way the students are expected to write an assessment, but if that is regarded as only being for the teacher practitioners' benefit, it may not help the students sufficiently to develop the habit of self-assessment
- a reflective journal is also becoming a common practice. The idea underlying this is that students are expected to keep a learning diary which may, or may not, form part of the formal assessment. Perhaps the classical case of this type of journal was the famous existentialist philosopher Gabriel Marcel (1976) who wrote *Being and Having* as a diary. Diaries can be used in a variety of different ways, for example, to identify critical learning incidents and comment on them, write a case/event from each day and analysis, etc.

It will be recalled that the learning cycle, discussed earlier in this book, has a stage of reflectivity and it is at this point that the teacher practitioners must encourage the students to reflect upon their practice and to learn from it, so that they are always endeavouring to improve their practice for the benefit of their clients/patients.

Conclusion

Teacher practitioners are, therefore, teachers, assessors and teachers of assessment techniques in order to encourage the students to develop the habit of self-assessment. In addition, they must be totally professional so that their practice, as teachers and practitioners, should also be open to their own self-appraisal. Yet there is a sense in which they are fortunate because, provided that they have developed good relationships with the students with whom they are working, they have colleagues who are able to comment upon their professional practice thereby helping them continue to improve the service they offer patients/clients and students. Since teacher practitioners have the opportunity to help the students, they should also be prepared to let the students help them improve and develop as part of the process of normal human interaction. The students will assess their teacher practitioners in any case, since this is natural in social interaction, so that the teacher practitioners may benefit considerably by encouraging the students to articulate their comments.

Thus far this text has concentrated quite specifically upon the teaching role of the teacher practitioner, but Chapter 7 widens the focus and examines the whole process of which teacher practitioners are but one part.

Perspectives on the educational process

7

This chapter explores:
- *Professional preparation*
- *The role performance of teacher practitioners and mentors*
- *The student's role.*

INTRODUCTION

The previous chapters of this book have examined the role of the teacher practitioner and mentor in terms of the educational process, but in this chapter the teacher practitioners' and mentors' roles are looked at from the broader perspective of the whole educational process.

PROFESSIONAL PREPARATION

The term preparation is used here in order to avoid the educational versus training debate – one which has occupied much space but produced little agreement over the years. Professional preparation refers to the whole process of preparing recruits for nursing, midwifery, health visiting and social work. This section opens with a brief discussion about the process of course preparation and validation, the aims and functions of professional preparation follow and, finally, the practical placement is examined.

COURSE PREPARATION AND VALIDATION

As a result of reorganization in recent years, a great deal of professional preparation has been located in higher education in the United Kingdom. For the most part those institutions of higher education have the authority to award their own qualifications, although some still seek validation from a more established institution of higher education, such as a chartered university. However, they still also require the approval of the professional body if their courses are to lead to professional recognition.

The normal process for an initial internal validation is for the course team to follow guidelines laid down by the higher education institution for the preparation of new courses. This usually involves preparing a validation document which includes information about the following:

- the reasons for the course – aims and objectives
- the location of the course within the mission of the educational institution
- the demand for the course
- contributing partners, such as health authorities
- the expectations of the professional body, for example, the relevant National Board for Nursing, Midwifery and Health Visiting and the Council for Education and Training of Social Workers, in order to gain professional recognition, where this is appropriate
- the funding arrangements and an approximate costing based on an optimum intake of students
- the course philosophy
- content
- teaching and learning strategies
- assessment procedures
- a draft timetable
- the teaching team and anticipated staff:student ratios
- teaching load and curricula vitae of all staff contributing to the course, and this might well include mentors and teacher practitioners
- course resources, for example, library and IT
- support in place for students, for example, counselling service
- expectations of the students
- draft student handbook
- outline curriculum for each module/theme, etc.
- arrangements for practical placements and assessment of practice
- quality control procedures and course evaluation
- grievance and appeal procedures
- the number of the external examiners and their role, including the frequency of meetings of the Board of Examiners.

It will be clear from the above list that teacher practitioners and mentors might be asked to play a significant part in the preparation of these validation documents. Depending upon their roles within the educational institution, the health authority or local authority, they will perform different functions in this process. However, many members of the course team will play a part in the formulation of the actual module or theme, each of which should include the following:

- the name of the course teacher/facilitator and other members of the course team contributing to the module, theme, etc.
- aims and objectives
- content and bibliography
- teaching/learning strategies
- methods of assessment and the value of the credit awarded
- amount of time allocated for the module/theme
- evaluation procedures.

Once the documents are prepared, they are submitted to the educational institution for validation for the institutional award, such as a degree or diploma, etc. Because of the professional nature of the courses, these documents must also be submitted to the professional body so that it can give its professional stamp of approval to the course, and allow successful students to be professionally recognized and, if applicable, have their names recorded on the professional register.

Some of the validation procedures are very thorough and often the validation body asks that its representatives should meet members of the course team, practitioners from placement areas and even students from other courses run by the institution, whose opinions are very important indeed. In addition, sometimes there are visits to professional placement sites. Consequently, teacher practitioners and mentors might be called on to assist both with the preparation of validation documents and, also, during the actual validation process itself.

The outcome of the validation process naturally depends upon how satisfied the validation committee is with what it has seen and heard during the process. The usual type of validation is for five years, occasionally for three and sometimes – especially if there is more work to be done on the submission – for one year with re-validation thereafter, etc. Sometimes, there is a complete rejection, but this is more unusual, since the course leader should have taken considerable soundings during the preparation process and the professional team should be sufficiently aware of the expectations to ensure that the submission is professionally and academically acceptable. To reduce the likelihood of rejection, some institutions actually run a mock validation exercise on their submission.

The validation process is part of the professional body's and the educational institution's quality assurance procedures and it is for this reason that the documentation has to be so full. In the event of a quality audit being conducted on the educational institution by the Higher Education Funding Council, this documentation may have to be produced. Nevertheless, it is a sign of the times and it is the quality of the documentation that is validated rather than the quality of the course! But in defence of this approach, the validation is really examining the ability, procedures and intentions of the course team to ensure that the course being offered is of an acceptable quality, and the actual course evaluation remains the responsibility of the course team and the educational institution.

THE AIMS OF PROFESSIONAL PREPARATION

Among the aims of preparing recruits for nursing, midwifery, health visiting and social work there is one specifying that new entrants to the profession should have the knowledge and skills to provide an excellent service. But it is also clear that to be a professional carer demands more than knowledge and skill, it demands sufficient commitment to render this service in a genuinely caring manner. However, it might be argued that the professional groups are seeking to indoctrinate recruits into their ideology if this were to be the aim of a course of professional preparation. But if sufficient commitment to providing a service is not an aim, then all the claims that the professions make about being caring professions would appear to be mere words. Hence, it should be an aim! But does this necessarily make it a process of indoctrination? Is it necessarily a process of inculcating acceptable attitudes into the new recruit? If the intention were to produce new entrants who believe every tenet of an occupational ideology of service then the accusation of indoctrination by intent would be justified. But there are many ways of rendering a service to patients/clients and there are many unique situations in which it is performed, so that conformity may not be intended – apart from the ideology of caring for all people irrespective of age, gender, colour, creed or race (Benner and Wrubel, 1989). Both illness and disability should be added to this list. It should be assumed that people who enter such professional preparation have that belief, but if they do not then their candidature should be rejected because they do not possess such a caring attitude. But should that specific attitude be taught during professional training? Professional preparation is about preparing people to care effectively rather than simply to care.

In these instances, the aims of professional preparation are not indoctrinational, especially as there should be another aim, that was discussed earlier in this book, which is to develop a critical attitude. Indeed, as these courses have moved into higher education, some scholars would argue that criticality is a fundamental feature of this form of education. Consequently, professional preparation in higher education should not only seek to produce knowledgeable and skilled practitioners, but also ones who are both caring and critical professionals.

FUNCTIONS OF PROFESSIONAL PREPARATION

The difference between aim and function is quite crucial to this discussion: an aim is a broad intention, but a function is the result of the implementation of the intention. In functionalist sociology the concept of function tended to mean the contribution the phenomenon made to the integration of the group, society, etc. Here, it is merely the results of professional preparation which may, but need not necessarily, be the same as the aims.

Perhaps the most obvious example of one of the functions of professional preparation is to be discovered in the procedures for selecting recruits for the profession. The candidate must have acquired a certain academic standard before she can be considered for entry and she must then undergo a selection procedure. There may be good reasons why nursing and social work wish to restrict their entry to those who have acquired a specific number of passes in the General Certificate of Secondary Education or the General Certificate of Education at Advanced Level, or for other branches of nursing, midwifery and health visiting to require other specific entry qualifications, but there is little empirical evidence to suggest that many of these arbitrary requirements actually relate to the ability to perform the professional role thereafter (Jarvis and Gibson, 1981). However, they do serve to prevent some people who have not acquired that standard from entry, even though they may have the potential to become efficient nurses or social workers. Every barrier to access creates a 'new poor', so that one of the functions of professional education is to select those who are considered acceptable to the profession. This selection function continues to operate in a variety of ways throughout the whole career of the nurse, but the teacher practitioner plays only a small part in the early stages. At the same time, it has to be recognized that many educational institutions do have alternative routes into professional courses, including ACCESS courses.

Another obvious function of professional education is that it enables the recruit to acquire sufficient knowledge and those skills and attitudes that the professions have decided are necessary before a recruit may be considered safe to enter practice. While the teaching and learning process may be seen as an overt one in which the tutor, the teacher practitioner and mentor play a significant part, there is a concurrent process of professional socialization. During this process the student is more covertly acquiring other attitudes that she recognizes as acceptable to the professions. In addition, the student is also acquiring a professional identity, so that she can say, 'I am a nurse . . .', 'I am a health visitor . . .' or I am a social worker . . .', etc. Simpson (1967) noticed how, during the professional socialization process, the service ethic of student nurses was transformed into a technical interest and the students' use of patients as significant others declined as they sought to acquire technical skills. Thereafter, the nurses began to acquire professional values as they were gradually crossing the divide between non-nurse and nurse and as they became accepted within the professional community. Teacher practitioners may witness some of these changes in the students with whom they work, especially if they work with them throughout the whole of their course.

Therefore, when these students enter their chosen occupation they will not disrupt the community of the professional group, so that another function of professional preparation is to ensure that there is continuity in the profession from one generation to the next, since those who have been trained, educated and socialized are able to assume their place in the profession without causing its structures any undue strain. However, it will be recalled that one of the aims of professional preparation is to create a sense of critical awareness in the students. If that aim were to be achieved to any great extent, then there is a possibility that critically-aware thinkers might prove a disruptive influence to the harmony of the profession, so that there is an inherent dysfunction in professional preparation. Nevertheless in this time of rapid social change, new ideas and new practices might prove beneficial to professional practice, so it is wise for experienced professionals to look carefully at the new ideas that recruits bring to their practice and to evaluate them in practice before rejecting them – it is in this way that teacher practitioners and mentors can actually learn from their students.

THE PRACTICAL PLACEMENT

In recent years, it has become very clear that professionals learn in practice (Schon, 1983; Krill, 1990; Baskett and Marsick, 1992). In addition, practical knowledge has become viewed as something much more significant than it was in previous generations when academic and theoretical knowledge was regarded as the most important acquisition of professional preparation. Consequently, the practical placement has assumed greater significance than ever before which means that the teacher practitioners' and mentors' roles are regarded more highly now than in the past.

It is in the practical placement that the teacher practitioners and mentors have opportunity of relating theory and practice, of showing students how to learn from practice situations and even how to theorize from them. It is also an opportunity for the students to develop their own frameworks for professional practice under guidance and with support. Here students learn how to criticize what they have learned, how to develop their own theoretical perspectives and, above all, how to perform in the professional practice situation. Student teachers, for example, build their own bodies of practical knowledge which they learn in and from practice and by adapting the theoretical knowledge that they have already learned in the classroom.

Here, under guidance, new recruits to the professions learn how to become practitioners; it is one of the major ways through which they acquire their professional identity and competence as a professional. It is here that the teacher practitioners and mentors perform a most valuable service.

THE ROLE PERFORMANCE OF TEACHER PRACTITIONERS AND MENTORS

This book commenced with an examination of the roles of the teacher practitioner and mentor and ends with a brief consideration of these roles. Each is a single, important occupational role in the context of preparing new recruits to nursing, midwifery, health visiting and social work. Throughout the book the theory and practice of teaching adults has been under consideration, irrespective of the actual occupation of the role player, since teaching adults is the common element. Teacher practitioners and mentors from the different branches of nursing and social work can themselves be prepared together because of the nature of this common element. To separate them is to the disservice of their common role, but to unite them is to acknowledge the centrality of their educational role and to enrich their learning experiences.

It is a role that the role players create for themselves and it is upon this assumption that this second part of the chapter focuses. It has six sections: understanding the role; creating relationships with students; the authority of the role; professionalism; reflective practice; self-evaluation.

UNDERSTANDING THE ROLE

In their own professional disciplines, teacher practitioners and mentors perform their own professional roles which are difficult and demanding, while at the same time they seek to be educators: they are both professional practitioners and professional educators of adults. The separation throughout this book has been for heuristic purposes only for, in point of fact, they are simultaneous and concurrent roles. But because it is a different role from that of other practitioners, there is a certain freedom to create their roles for themselves, although it is still circumscribed by the demands of the course of which they are an integral part. At the same time, they interact with a wide variety of people as they play that role – this is their role set.

Merton (1968 pp41–5) has argued that individuals perform their roles differently as they interact with the different people in the role set. The implications of this are that if all the members of the role set have certain expectations of the way that the role should be played, it is difficult for the role player to resist the social pressures to conform. However, if there is a diversity of attitudes among the role set, then there is some freedom for the role player to negotiate the way that they perform their role. There is, therefore, more flexibility in the way that the role is performed and so it approximates to the autonomous approach to role performance that many people seek.

However, the education of adults is a young discipline and most people's attitudes to teaching and learning might still be coloured by their own experience in school or in their initial occupational preparation. Hence, it would not be difficult to envisage a situation in which the expectations that some members of the role set have about the teacher practitioner's or mentor's role performance do not appear to be in accord with their own. Imagine an instance in which a nurse manager thinks that the learner-centred approach allows the student too much latitude; the tutor wishes the teacher practitioner to follow a prescribed syllabus; the student wants the teacher practitioner to be more teacher-centred; colleagues feel that the approach needs to be more tightly structured: what should the teacher practitioner do? Clearly constant pressure might force her to conform to a more teacher-centred approach. But if that is the case, then cultural reproduction may be perpetuated and the teacher practitioner might still be an instructor rather than a teacher of adults. It is in instances such as this that associations of teacher practitioners and mentors are important, since members can provide support for each other in their role performance.

The picture drawn in the previous paragraph may not depict reality at all and, by contrast, teacher practitioners and mentors may gain support from all the members of their role set, so that they do not have to explain and negotiate with each of the members. Even so, it is the teacher practitioner's and mentor's responsibility to decide how they should play their role, within the prescribed parameters of the Health Service and the educational institution, but since she does work in a team, it may always be necessary to explain why she is using the approach that she does. By creating her own role, the teacher practitioner or mentor may construct something that is uniquely theirs, and as such is most satisfying to perform.

CREATING HUMAN RELATIONSHIPS

It has been maintained, from the outset, that in the individualized teaching and learning interaction it is vitally important that a harmonious relationship is established between the teacher practitioner and the student. Such a relationship cannot be established if teacher practitioners or mentors seek to be authoritarian, even though their positions do give them some responsibilities.

The significance of the relationship between teacher practitioners and mentors and their students is the maximization of the student's learning that was discussed earlier in this study. This is a process of human interaction in which it is assumed that both partners wish to achieve a harmonious relationship, but that the roles that they play are open to negotiation. Hence, the actors will be seeking to act in accordance with the way that they perceive the other expects them to perform, so that they will both be seeking symbolic expressions from the other to guide them. They will adapt their role in accordance with the symbols that are perceived in order to achieve a norm. Clearly the teacher practitioners and mentors may have to take the lead in this process since there are status differences that would prevent many students from so doing. Moreover, the symbols that are manifest are not only those that the actors know that they are giving (for example, the spoken words, the smile), but there are other symbols 'given off' which may be less conscious and less intended but which will also be received by the other person in the relationship and interpreted accordingly. Not only are the two actors giving and receiving symbols about how they should interact with each other, it must also be borne in mind that they come from different backgrounds and bring their own wealth of experiences with them to the interaction. Hence, they each have their own sub-cultural differences and these have to be negotiated, so that there is a sense in which their meeting provides an arena for the negotiation of these disparities.

Despite these differences, it has to be recognized that all people are created equal in respect of their humanity, even if they have neither similar abilities nor advantages, and in the individualized teaching and learning situation a relationship is not established by exercise of hierarchical position nor manifestation of unequal abilities but, rather, it is established upon the humanity of the participants. In this relationship two human beings bring together their own humanity and their experiences: it is a relationship of equal adult human beings, with the self of each being of infinite value which is to be treasured and nurtured within the social intercourse. Anything occurring within that relationship that threatens the dignity of either participant or the development of the other's self may be considered immoral. Indeed, Levinas (1991 p43) has cogently argued that when another calls into question an actor's spontaneity, there is the beginning of ethics (see Jarvis, 1977, for a fuller exposition of this argument). The point is that the relationship which is formed between teacher practitioners or mentors and their students is necessarily a moral one. Indeed, at the very heart of the role performance lies an ethical relationship which actually transcends the professional codes of ethics. It is imperative that the participants respect each other's humanity and that the teacher practitioners and mentors seek to create and develop such relationships.

THE AUTHORITY OF TEACHER PRACTITIONERS AND MENTORS

Authority is not intrinsic to the person, it is either attributed because of position or because of the knowledge or skill that a person possesses. The former authority is dependent totally upon the relationship between the individuals and the organization in which they are employed; it is ascribed without necessarily having been earned, so that while the office holder may have her authority obeyed, she may not necessarily command respect. Teacher practitioners and mentors are usually senior persons within the service and, as such, they hold positions of responsibility; they are teachers and managers, etc., and the positions do not only carry certain responsibilities, they also carry certain privileges and rewards. Such differentiation of roles, responsibilities and privileges is considered by some to be necessary in contemporary society for it to function effectively, although too much differentiation in rewards and privileges opens itself to questions of morality.

Naturally, as senior employees this authority of position exists, but this should not be the type of authority by which teacher practitioners and mentors expect to conduct their relationship with their students and mentees. They should seek the latter form of authority, that bestowed upon them because of their expertise as practitioners and/or as teachers and mentors. In this instance, the practitioners have earned the authority and are respected for what they know and can do; this is not the kind of authority that can be written down and institutionalized, but it is the authority of the professional.

PROFESSIONALISM

Throughout the text professionalism has been viewed as an ideology of endeavouring to be the master of the discipline in order to render service of the highest kind to the client/patient. Such mastery is not for the purpose of self-aggrandizement but in order to be of service. Failure to be the master means that ultimately the practitioner does not really care sufficiently for those who are being served to undertake the hard work and the continuing learning necessary to remain an expert. Hence she ceases to be professional, because she does not care sufficiently to give the best service to her fellow human beings and so she fails to respect their humanity.

The morality of professionalism rests, then, upon the motivation to provide a quality service and it is this that teacher practitioners and mentors should both exhibit themselves and also seek to ensure that those whom they teach and mentor also demonstrate. Teacher practitioners and mentors cannot expect their learners and mentees to demonstrate professionalism unless they themselves manifest it. However, if the learner or mentee fails to demonstrate a professional attitude during preparation it is maintained here that this constitutes sufficient reason for teacher practitioners and mentors to recommend some form of deferment when they submit their report to the Board of Examiners; obviously such a decision should not come as a surprise to the student or mentee since the teacher practitioners or mentors should have already discussed the problem with the student and tried to help her to overcome it prior to making such a recommendation.

In recent years, the term professional has taken second place to expert in much of the literature (Benner, 1984) and this is probably because a great deal of the concerns about professional lay with the body of professional knowledge rather than the expertise to practise. Certainly, there was an over-emphasis on knowledge to the detriment of practitioner expertise, but professionals should be as expert practitioners as they are possessors of professional knowledge.

It is recognized, however, that as the bodies of knowledge in nursing, midwifery, health visiting and social work and in the education of adults increases, this creates major problems for busy teacher practitioners and mentors. Clearly they are expected to be expert practitioners in both elements of their work and, also, to be familiar with two bodies of knowledge. It is this which makes these roles extremely demanding and one which suggests that before professional expertise is attained, something Benner (1984 pp20–34) suggests takes a number of years, the teaching and mentoring role should not be undertaken. Teacher practitioners and mentors have to be experts and professionals in both strands of their role.

REFLECTIVE PRACTITIONERS

All learning stems from experience, so it was argued earlier in this book. This means that practice is as much a site for learning as is the classroom. Teacher practitioners and mentors will be expected to help their students and mentees become reflective practitioners, but part of this process is through setting an example – by being a reflective practitioner. All practice provides opportunity for practitioners, however experienced they are, to learn from practice – both as practitioners and as teachers or mentors. But, like most busy professionals, the 'busyness' of everyday life does tend to get in the way and many potential learning situations become non-learning ones. Consequently, it is incumbent on all who undertake the responsible task of helping junior colleagues to ensure that they themselves are always endeavouring to keep abreast with developments in the field, always learning from practice and, even more importantly, always being prepared to problematize situations which become taken-for-granted situations so that new learning opportunities arise.

This responsibility is the teacher practitioners' or mentors', but where educational or other employing organizations allocate this role to experienced professionals, they also have a responsibility to ensure that these learning and reflecting periods are also built into the job descriptions. In the current situation where both education and the Health Service operate in market economies, and managers often expect too much from their most experienced employees, they have sometimes to forego the demands of so-called economic efficiency for the sake of quality, and allow those who try to straddle two professions opportunity to reflect on both and to develop their own expertise in practice.

SELF-EVALUATION OF ROLE PERFORMANCE

Teacher practitioners and mentors should be professional and, as was discussed in Chapter 6, should constantly assess their role performance as they play it with each member of their role set. Self-assessment should make them aware of their own learning needs and their professionalism should drive them on to become self-directed learners. The students who work with them may be the only people who observe their role performance with all members of the role set and, provided that the relationship that has been established between them is harmonious, their comments may be useful and beneficial to help them continue to evaluate their own role performance. For as long as they assess and re-assess that role performance they will remain professional and once the critical awareness of self-assessment disappears then their professionalism is in danger of being compromised. Continual self-evaluation is one of the hallmarks of the professional, leading to more learning, and the enthusiasm to learn is one of those attitudes that should be transmitted in the process of professional socialization, so that the best service can be rendered to the patient or client.

THE STUDENT'S ROLE

Now the student's, or mentee's, role is examined in two sections: the first looks at learning to be a student and the second examines student grievance and appeal procedures.

LEARNING TO BE A STUDENT OR MENTEE IN THE PRACTICAL PLACEMENT

It will have become clear that the way that the student's, or mentee's, role is performed is a little different from that which many students who have come through a traditional educational process would expect. Many might come to their teacher practitioners or mentors not knowing precisely how to behave, or what to expect. In precisely the same way that many educational institutions are now running courses helping students to use a wider range of media for studying, it is useful for teacher practioners and mentors to do something similar for their students or mentees, in order to reinforce this process. Teacher practitioners and mentors will have their own expectations of the students and mentees, so it is wise, during the initial stages of working together, for the students to be given opportunity of negotiating their role with their teacher practitioners or mentors, of finding out precisely what is expected of them, etc. This is not a matter of the teacher practitioners or mentors laying down precise rules and regulations, or even precise expectations, but it is a matter of helping students and mentees begin to learn how to play their adult, professional student role in the practical situation. It is a matter of having boundaries and understandings, a matter of knowing something about expectations and role behaviour, etc. Having entered into an informal contract, students and mentees will feel much more at ease in their role and relationships. Indeed, freedom is often more easy to practise when the framework has been laid than when the students and mentees are never sure what is expected of them or what are the boundaries of the relationship, etc.

GRIEVANCE AND APPEAL PROCEDURES

Every course will have its own grievance and appeal procedures which are usually published in the student handbook for the course. In the same way, health authorities have their own published grievance procedures. These procedures should be readily available to all members of the course, both staff and students, so that students may know their rights and staff respond to grievance or appeals in a correct manner. Teacher practitioners and mentors (where appropriate) should acquaint themselves with these procedures so that they can advise their students about the appropriate procedures, if unfortunate circumstances arise. If, however, the grievance or an appeal is about the teacher practitioner or mentor, then it is advisable for them to stand back from the relationship and let others undertake all aspects of the enquiry. It appears that grievances and appeals are being enacted more frequently in the present times than is past times, so it is always wise for teacher practitioners and mentors to keep fairly full records of all the dealings with students and mentees, which might provide the necessary evidence if such unfortunate circumstances should arise. They should always be able to justify their position in respect of either a grievance or an appeal.

Conclusion

This chapter has begun to explore some other perspectives on the education and training of professionals. It has endeavoured to locate it in the wider world of higher education but, as Chapter 8 will demonstrate, even this is undergoing rapid social changes and is being influenced by forces that have not previously played a significant part in this educational process. In addition, it demonstrates how the current emphasis on the practical and on practical knowledge is itself a sign of the times.

Contemporary reflections on the educational process

8

This chapter explores:
- *The changing nature of knowledge*
- *The changing nature of education*
- *The teacher practitioner in the late modern society.*

INTRODUCTION

This final chapter seeks to locate the processes discussed earlier in the book within the much wider context of the changes that are occurring within education generally. This is significant since the professional preparation of social workers, nurses, midwives and health visitors has been incorporated within higher education. Indeed, it is even more apposite when it is recognized that postmodern scholars are suggesting that knowledge is being legitimated by its performability (Lyotard, 1984) – that is, that the basis for the legitimation of knowledge is its practicality.

This chapter assumes a meta-theoretical stance, examining theoretical knowledge rather than practical knowledge, so that teacher practitioners and mentors may see their role against the broader backcloth of the academic disciplines as well as social work, nursing, midwifery and health visiting.

THE CHANGING NATURE OF KNOWLEDGE

Modernity, a cultural phenomenon of Western society which emerged with the Enlightenment, is typified by an emphasis on scientific knowledge, empiricism, rationality, universality, individualism, secularism and progress. As a result of the Enlightenment, Western society reflected these values at a time when its power was dominant and its culture regarded as having reached the apex of civilization. Indeed, the discourse of Modernity contained these assumptions. These were also the values embraced by the intellectuals who were, to some extent, the guardians of a culture supporting the power of the modern state. As a result, education played a significant role in the development of modern society.

All of the professions, almost without exception, endeavoured to formulate their knowledge base in these scientific terms. Social work, nursing, midwifery and health visiting have been no exception, although in more recent times this 'scientific' base of knowledge has been questioned by postmodern scholars. This has meant that claims to be scientific may be treated with a little more scepticism than previously.

Indeed, the nature of knowledge itself has undergone profound changes, with four major ones being suggested here. Knowledge is now regarded as: relative (almost narrative); its rational basis has changed; its modes of transmission have altered; it has become a marketable commodity.

THE RELATIVITY OF KNOWLEDGE

When Lyotard (1984) wrote *The Post-Modern Condition* he claimed that all knowledge had become narrative, but later he (1992 p31) recognized that he had over-emphasized his position and he then suggested that different forms of knowledge had to be recognized, even though he still considered many forms of knowledge to be narrative. It must also be noted that as globalization has occurred there is an increase in relativism. The point about a great deal of the previous discourse is that it reflected the dominant theories of the day and, as is now widely recognized, the prevailing received knowledge does appear to change with great rapidity.

The question might well be posed about the extent to which there is unchanging scientific knowledge, and clearly nobody is going to reject the idea that there are some universal and unchanging laws of nature, although it must be recognized that these occur with much less frequency than it was previously claimed. Advances in scientific research do tend to modify prevailing theories and this has also come to be rather taken for granted; new discoveries reveal more about phenomena than was previously known; new technological advances mean that what was impossible a year or two ago now becomes possible and becomes an everyday occurrence tomorrow. Scientific knowledge, therefore, has become recognized as relative and its validity can always be questioned as other evidence is produced to refute or recast a current theory. Academics who previously legislated on what was correct knowledge have now become interpreters in a world of new knowledge (Bauman, 1992b) and, perhaps, legitimators of learning.

Other disciplines, such as the social sciences, have tried to be scientific in their approach and as they have approximated to the scientific, they have discovered that there are myths regarding the claims about the nature of scientific knowledge itself. Indeed, it is perhaps significant that the terms learning and information are sometimes preferred to knowledge, since the latter term implies a finitude, or an end-product, while the former one suggest that that which is known is only partial and that the progress of discovery is incomplete.

THE RATIONAL BASIS OF KNOWLEDGE

The birth of Modernity brought with it an increasing emphasis on empiricism at the time of the Enlightenment. The traditional narratives about the world were being destroyed by the scientific discoveries and rational arguments of the age. The then new universities grew up in this age of Modernity, often with the express intention of disseminating this new scientific knowledge to an eager population. University extramural lectures emerged during this period with reports of many hundreds of people coming to lectures about recent scientific discoveries. Knowledge was regarded as empirically true and, therefore, valid. Empiricism was regarded as the basis of a great deal of this new knowledge and those who discovered it were the legislators of what was correct. The universities were in a position to pronounce on what was correct and true knowledge, and the professions wanted, or needed, to be associated with them.

But now the basis of knowledge is changing. Increasingly it is becoming apparent that many statements about society are ideological rather than empirical, and claims about it seen to be discourse rather than factual. These may still be firmly based in reason, although they are harder to substantiate. Indeed, there has also been an increase in narratives about what society should be like, rather than what it is – more ethical studies and even a return to utopian studies (for example, Kumar, 1987; Levitas, 1990).

But there is another basis to knowledge that it now being accepted and this is clearly described by Lyotard (1984 p48), who argues that the knowledge that the universities teach is now only socially legitimated by the criterion of the performability in the social system, so that they have to produce skilled experts since:

> The transmission of knowledge is no longer destined to train an elite capable of guiding the nation towards its emancipation, but to supply the system with players capable of acceptably fulfilling their roles at the pragmatic posts required by the institution.

He goes on to argue that once knowledge ceases to be an end in itself, its transmission is no longer the exclusive responsibility of scholars and students. Knowledge is now based on pragmatism. This is not the place to explore the philosophy of pragmatism, although it might be claimed now that knowledge is legitimated by its utility. If something works, then it can be transmitted to others. However, the issue is perhaps deeper than this since universities are being urged to seek research funding from industry and commerce – the knowledge being produced is based on its perceived utility. Once produced, it needs to be transmitted to those who need it, so that another new concept has become quite central to universities and colleges in recent years: namely, continuing education. Continuing education used to be called adult education and then there was a combination of terms such as adult and continuing education, and now the adult has been dropped from much common usage and continuing education has become the accepted term. People need continuing education so that they can continue in their work and develop both professionally and personally. Indeed, it is now expected of many professional groups, including nursing and midwifery, and for some it is necessary in order to continue on the professional register. The English National Board (1995) has also facilitated the introduction of continuing education courses which lead to specialist practitioner qualifications. Universities are also being increasingly asked to conduct an impact evaluation on what they are teaching, that is the performance outcome in the organization from which the students come. To a great extent, the validity of continuing education is pragmatic – that is, it is performable – since its value depends on its impact on society. The philosophy of pragmatism, however, does need to be revisited.

As we have seen in this book, the re-emergence of the concept of practical knowledge is significant in this respect, for practical knowledge is not discipline-based but practice-based. Neither education nor nursing can ever be regarded as academic disciplines, but they are fields of practice, for example, there can be a sociology of education and a philosophy of nursing, but there cannot be an education of sociology nor a nursing of philosophy. Practical education knowledge is multi-disciplinary and so is practical nursing knowledge. In a real sense, in practical knowledge there are no barriers between the academic disciplines.

TRANSMISSION OF KNOWLEDGE

At the birth of Modernity, there were basically two modes of knowledge transmission, spoken and written, and the universities were undertaking both. The lecture theatre was the locus for the transmission of learning and the publishing houses, with such illustrious names as Oxford and Cambridge, being the other major mode of knowledge transmission. When wireless became the third major mode, the

universities were notably absent, as they were with the birth of tele-
vision. Eventually, with the birth of the Open University in the
United Kingdom, the universities reclaimed a place in the modern mode
of knowledge transmission. Clearly, the Open University was, and
continues to be, a great success and its knowledge production is of a
Fordist nature – mass production for a mass market, with some courses
prepared for 100,000 students. Significantly, questions are now being
raised about post-Fordist methods of production, and perhaps there is
a place here for the modern university in this late modern world
of learning.

Yet the world has moved on since 1970, and now it is an information
society and there are institutions like the Fielding Institute in America
which does not use printed materials at all – the electronic university
is a reality. But the electronic university is but one stage in this transformation. Now there are the Internet, satellites, cable TV and compact
discs, and this is not just one-way transmission, and the possibilities of
interactive media are also here. Indeed, some commercial companies are
already producing interactive video compact discs, so that knowledge
can be taught and learned interactively, and cable has even more potential. The research and development costs of these innovations have been
considerable, so it could hardly be expected that a single university
could produce such material – although Associated Universities, a
commercial company in Tennessee sponsored by a number of universities, has been producing technological learning material under contract
for many years.

KNOWLEDGE AS A MARKETABLE COMMODITY

Knowledge, then, can now be packaged and marketed. In the information society, this information might not now be called teaching materials,
but learning packages, or learning materials, both of which have now
become familiar terms. This is an information-led society and knowledge has become a commodity that can be sold, like any other. However,
it is even more important than many of the products on the market.
Lyotard (1984 p5) wrote:

> Knowledge in the form of an informational commodity indis-
> pensable to productive power is already, and will continue to be,
> a major – perhaps the major – stake in the worldwide competition
> for power. It is conceivable that nation-states will one day fight
> for control of information, just as they battled in the past for control
> over territory.

National states, however, are themselves subject to intense pressures
with the process of globalization, so it might be conglomerate states or

transnational companies that battle with each other. Universities and colleges which purvey information are now part of an extensive and complex scene in which they are rarely the largest players. Indeed, the transnational companies that are able to invest millions of dollars in the research and production of these means of transmitting knowledge are also able to invest the same amount of capital in the research and development of knowledge itself. They are able to produce their own learning materials and market them.

Educational institutions still, to a large extent, rely on local and instantaneous transmission of knowledge, i.e. the learners have to be present when the lecture is delivered, although they are slowly moving to other forms of open and distance learning, but the new market has both space–time distanciation (Giddens, 1990) and, in the information society, space–time compression (Harvey, 1989): knowledge can be transmitted and learned not at the teachers' convenience but at the learners', and that this can be done worldwide and instantaneously since the market is now global, etc.

Information, then, is an important, relative commodity that is being marketed by many different organizations. The basis of knowledge in society has changed and become more pragmatic, and its culture is one where there are ample opportunities to acquire such learning packages. Having examined the way that knowledge is changing, it is now important to examine the ways that this is already affecting and will continue to affect higher education, of which nursing, health visiting, midwifery and social work education is a part.

THE CHANGING NATURE OF EDUCATION

Clearly these changes are having profound effects on education, and will have even more profound effects on higher education in the future. Five aspects will be discussed here: higher education; education and learning; vocational and leisure time learning; the learners; the nature of the dissemination of information.

HIGHER EDUCATION

Universities used to be very distinct and they were for the elite, but with the changing nature of knowledge, the universities are losing their distinctive place in society. Now there is a need, not for an educated elite, but for an highly educated technological workforce and this could comprise as much as 30 per cent of the total working population. Reich calls these the symbolic analysts; the other two groups are in-person services and routine production services (Reich, 1991). This means that universities have to cater for a far larger proportion of the population than ever before, and so more universities are created and university education becomes a system of mass higher education. Professional groups like nursing, midwifery, health visiting and social work are among the many new occupations finding their place in this new world of higher education (see de Wit, 1993 pp10–11).

However, the symbolic analysts need continual updating, leading to continuing education, and so more higher taught degrees are beginning to appear. As the more established universities concentrate on post-graduate degrees, so they franchise their lower degree work to colleges of further and higher education and institutes of higher education. The boundaries between higher education and further education are, therefore, becoming more and more blurred.

EDUCATION AND LEARNING

For a long time educators have confused the terms education and learning; indeed, they have treated them as synonymous. Hence, it has been hard to distinguish between the use of adult education and adult learning, and lifelong education and lifelong learning, etc. What is now happening is that the distinction between these two ideas is becoming clearer. Learning is something which people do, while education is a social institution which provides learning opportunities for people. The significance of this is that, with the advent of the information society, a great deal of learning material is becoming more easily available to individuals, often at a market price, but that the providers need not be organizations which are commonly regarded as educational. An individual can undertake a course of learning which has been purchased in a retail outlet or attend classes in the same subject at a local adult educational institution. In the one instance, it is learning and the other it might be considered to be educational. The crucial difference at the present time is the nature of the provider rather than the mode of dissemination or the subject studied. The significance of the above illustration is that it is the same subject being studied – the choice of provider is now with the learner. This is part of the nature of the change – the learner might choose to purchase the learning from an educational institution or from another provider of learning materials. This is already occurring in nursing, and it can be confidently expected that the process will continue as the learning market plays a more significant role in education.

VOCATIONAL AND LEISURE TIME LEARNING

People can learn throughout the length and breadth of their lives, for both work and leisure. The whole of life is a potential learning arena, which has often been crudely separated into two: a vocational and a leisure time pursuit. Leisure time learning can involve any subject that is of interest to the learner. Similarly, vocational education refers to every occupation, so there are many different fields of practice and it is almost impossible to chart them all. Indeed, as the world becomes more complex, the boundaries between leisure time and vocational learning are becoming even more blurred.

The knowledge explosion has resulted in the need for some occupations to introduce regular updating for their members in order to ensure that they are reasonably abreast with the latest thinking – the UKCC requires nurses, health visitors and midwives to undertake regular updating in order to remain on the professional register – so that there has been a massive growth in continuing vocational education over the past few years. Indeed, as early as 1960, Kerr *et al.* suggested that education is the handmaiden of industry and that only those subjects useful to industry should be included in the curriculum – all other subjects should be regarded as leisure time activities. They (Kerr *et al.*, 1973 p47) recognize precisely what type of educational system will emerge:

> Such an educational system is not primarily concerned with conserving traditional values or perpetuating the classics;

However, they were really only concerned about higher education when they expressed this view. Vocational continuing education has become pre-eminent and adult leisure time education is wrongly regarded as something of a historical anachronism. The fact that many people learn for learning's sake is a well-known phenomenon in adult education – this is leisure time learning. Kerr *et al.* recognized this and suggested that the arts and humanities, which were of apparently little vocational value in the industrial society, should constitute the curriculum for leisure time learning.

THE LEARNERS

Clearly in a world of rapid social change everybody has to respond to the change and so everybody is a learner. Therefore, the retail companies selling their learning materials will undertake their own market research to discover their potential market. People, because of the changes that they experience, are now aware of the need to learn to a greater extent than ever before.

Those who enrol in courses in educational institutions are the learners who have been the traditional focus of research in the education of adults. Sargant (1990) conducted a major survey in the United Kingdom in which she showed that 10 per cent of adults were currently engaged in studying and a further 16 per cent had studied in the previous three years. She also found that 10 per cent more were consciously undertaking self-directed learning, and this is the figure which is likely to rise as more multi-media learning packages are produced.

Sargant also found that a high proportion of men received vocational education, whereas more women were engaged in leisure time education. However, the growth of elder learning might well begin to change these figures in the coming years. It is clear that education for elders is an increasingly common phenomenon, with Elderhostel, University of the Third Age and even folk high schools especially devoted to seniors.

NATURE OF THE DISSEMINATION OF LEARNING OPPORTUNITIES

It was mentioned earlier in this chapter that the global society has seen two re-alignments of time and space, space–time distanciation (Giddens, 1990) and space–time compression (Harvey, 1989). Both of these are significant for the ways in which education and learning opportunities are developing.

Traditionally, education has been conducted at a point where space and time intersect. Learners have to be where the teachers are and so teacher–student interaction occurs. This form of education is clearly important and will not be phased out as a result of these changes, although even changes in the way this is conducted might occur. For instance, since teaching is an expensive commodity, it might be that the best teacher–learner ratios will occur in non-formal educational settings, such as the University of the Third Age, where the teachers are not paid. In addition, this will also occur in highly specialized areas, where the teacher is a specialist and few people could perform the same role in the same subject. However, this latter instance will be an expensive process and will occur less frequently. In addition, a new phenomenon might occur with teaching packages being prepared which are then taught by less well qualified teachers, so that the same course can be taught a number of times by different assistants during its shelf life. It will be rather like teaching assistants in schools but, in this case, the courses could actually be purchased by educational providers and taught – a form of enfranchisement. This approach is clearly possible with the type of space–time compression which has resulted in short modules, thus allowing for a change of learning menu whenever the learner desires to explore a new topic area.

Space–time compression has also resulted in new forms of delivery, such as fax, e-mail, satellite, cable and the Internet, so that it is now possible to study courses that are transmitted from any part of the world, and even have tutorials across the globe. Courses already exist on the world-wide web and the virtual university is in the process of being created.

Space–time distanciation has already meant that traditional distance education courses have separated the teacher/writer of the learning material from the learners. It is possible, through all forms of transmission, to study courses years after they are produced and for educational, and other, institutions to continue to market courses long after the authors of the course have left the institution, provided that the course is still marketable. Some courses might still be marketed beyond their 'sell-by' date, but this would be immoral unless they had been updated.

Clearly, the providers for all this material do not have to be only educational institutions because many other agencies involved in transmitting knowledge are able to undertake the same process. There is now a market for learning materials, one which might become even more competitive. However, the market is a complex phenomenon – it is not just a matter of supply and demand, which is the rationality of modernity and one which does not reflect the realities of a late modern society. Marketing is about selling brand names and signs. Indeed, Baudrillard (cited in Prosser 1988 p22) highlights this in his discussion of consumption in *The System of Objects*:

> Consumption is *the virtual totality of all objects and message presently constituted in a more or less coherent discourse*. Consumption, in so far as it is meaningful, is *a systematic act of the manipulation of signs*.
> (Italics in the original)

Baudrillard has argued that for phenomena to become objects of consumption, they must become signs. It is at this point that the educational system currently has a great advantage over other purveyors of learning – it has an established and widely recognized system of signs, which are the educational qualifications. Educational qualifications demonstrate that the learning which has been undertaken is legitimate and that it is recognized as such. The qualification has become a currency in the market for occupation, and possession of such a qualification demonstrates that the individual has the necessary learning to undertake the work. But jobs are changing and becoming more complex, and knowledge, since it is relative, is rapidly dated by new discoveries. Additional signs are required by the market to show that potential candidates for work have the recent knowledge necessary to undertake the work. Qualifications become outdated and new ones are required. A new phenomenon is emerging – qualification inflation, for example, certificates are replaced by diplomas; the Bachelors degree and then the Masters degree become devalued and the taught doctorate is becoming the new sign of a well-qualified professional. This could be seen as part of the process of professionalizing, although such an interpretation is rather unrealistic in this complex and rapidly changing world.

Educational institutions, therefore, can legitimate learning throughout the whole of life. At the present moment, educational institutions and professional associations hold a near-monopoly in the United Kingdom when it comes to legitimating learning, but the question has to be asked, How long this will continue? Already there are commercial organizations which award their own qualifications. As Eurich (1985 p85) notes:

> A new development on the scene of business and education is the growing number of corporate colleges, institutes, or universities that grant their own degrees. It is the Rand Ph.D., the Wang or Arthur D. Little Master of Science degree. No longer the purview of established educational institutions alone, accredited academic degrees are being awarded increasingly by companies and industries that have created their own separate institutions and successfully passed the same educational hurdles used to accredit traditional higher education.

This development, which has already started in the United Kingdom in a co-operative manner, might well develop in the way that Eurich suggests, so it might not be long before corporate institutions are marketing cultural knowledge and legitimating it through the award of their own qualifications. This is the logical development of what is currently occurring in the educational market and adults are much more easily able to purchase their learning materials on the open market – although people on low incomes will once again be disadvantaged, as they always are with the market economy, and this could lead to a re-emergence of radical forms of adult education.

Educational institutions will have to discover that there are niche markets and that the relativity of modern knowledge is not conducive to Fordist modes of production, so in a post-Fordist age of production they have a significant role to play, albeit in co-operation with other providers.

Thus it may be seen that learning materials are being and will continue to be, disseminated by a variety of means and this change is paradigmatic in education, so that it is becoming increasingly important to explore the research agenda for educators of adults.

THE TEACHER PRACTITIONER IN THE LATE MODERN SOCIETY

It will be seen from the above discussion that both the nature of knowledge and the nature of education are undergoing quite profound changes. Much of this discussion provides a theoretical underpinning for the work of teacher practitioners and mentors, and four points are highlighted here: the practical nature of knowledge; the new emphasis in education on learning from practical experience; the place of mentors and teacher practitioners in new forms of educational provision; the need for continuing education for the symbolic analysts.

THE PRACTICAL NATURE OF KNOWLEDGE

It will be clear from the above discussion that both knowledge and education are changing rapidly. The emphasis being placed upon practical knowledge reflects the form of knowledge which constitutes the teacher practitioner's and mentor's own role. It is a teaching role based in practice. But it is more than this, it is a form of knowledge driven by the demands of practice, which obviates the old theory–practice dichotomy.

In Chapter 1 we made a clear distinction between 'being able' and 'practical knowledge'. But we know that when we perform a procedure and it does not work out in the way that we expected, then we ask 'Why?' Why did this not occur in the way that we expected it to? We then have to look at the situation, examine the experience and learn from it – as the learning diagram in Chapter 4 illustrated. Having analyzed the situation, we might evolve new knowledge or a new skill as a result of the analysis, and we can then try them out in practice. If they work for the situation, then we can accept them until they fail and then the process begins again. The point about every practice situation, as Heller (1984: 168) points out, is that 'everything we do ... is based on probability'. Professionals act on sufficient grounds – their knowledge and expertise. The point is that both the new knowledge and the new skill evolve from the situation. In other words, they are practice-driven and the pragmatic relationship denotes something of the unity of practice and theory.

Now this is directly opposed to having a theory and seeking to apply it to practice. As Schon (1983) argued, technical rationality is dead. But the significance of this is even greater since for many decades scholars and practitioners have argued over the theory–practice divide. Now, there is no divide, for the new knowledge evolves from the practice and integrates the two in practical knowledge. The practical assumes new significance and, as Lyotard (1984) argued, the knowledge is legitimated by its performability.

LEARNING FROM PRACTICAL EXPERIENCE

Clearly, the significance of the experiential learning perspective adopted in Chapter 4 might now be recognized. Practical knowledge can be taught in the classroom, but learning how to do something can only occur in practice. The knowledge taught in the classroom can only be legitimated for practitioners when they learn, from the primary experience of practice, the extent to which the practical knowledge that they learned through secondary experiences in the classroom is valid.

Having learned practical knowledge in the classroom in a theoretical sense, practitioners can only identify with it when they have actually undertaken the procedures and practised it, and learned that they are both able to do it and that they actually do know how to do it.

Teacher practitioners and mentors have an important role of being with the learners when they are experimenting and seeing whether they can actually make some practical knowledge learned in the classroom their own through practice. It is also in practice that other new situations emerge and learners are exposed to new experiences that they can also learn from experimentation, using their previous knowledge and skills, etc. (their biography) in new ways. Sometimes, these new experiences may be facilitated by teacher practitioners and mentors.

It is in all of these situations that learners may need the help and support of mentors and teacher practitioners. For now practice is seen as a major learning site for professional practitioners, and learning theory is rightly focusing upon the experiences from which individuals learn rather than the more limiting theories of conditioning which emerged from the work of Pavlov and Skinner (for example, the studies of the times that dogs salivate or the ways by which rats and pigeons find their ways to food).

THE PLACE OF MENTORS AND TEACHER PRACTITIONERS

It will be clear from the previous sub-section that mentors and teacher practitioners have an important role complementing that of the classroom teacher. However, it was argued earlier in this chapter that new technology and harsh economics are moving education away from the expensive luxury of teaching in space–time instantiation. Now new forms of distance learning are individualizing learning and enabling theoretical learning to take place through interactive compact video disc and many other electronic media. This aspect of learning is certainly going to increase and as it is discovered that professional education can be cheaper through using these techniques, there will be an inevitable decline in classroom teaching. Despite the increase in simulations, actual learning how to perform a procedure with a live client can only occur in practice! It is only with the help and support of teacher practitioners and mentors that many learner practitioners will acquire the confidence and some of the skills to introduce new techniques into their practice, from which they can make the new knowledge their own. Consequently, the roles of teacher practitioner and mentor become more important with the growth and development of new forms of dissemination of professional knowledge.

THE GROWTH OF CONTINUING EDUCATION

The rapidity in the speed of knowledge change means that there will always be a demand for continuing education. With it, there will be a growth in professional qualifications and grade inflation as more and more practitioners seek masters degrees and, thereafter, practitioner doctorates for, as Lyotard (1984) pointed out, this practical knowledge is now needed for the practitioners, the symbolic analysts. Consequently institutions of further and higher education will concentrate even more upon professional practitioners as a major part of their student body. For as long as knowledge continues to change with this rapidity, continuing learning will be necessary for practitioners, especially in this age of litigation. Continuing learning and education are fundamentally practical and so many of those who teach will need to be expert practitioners themselves. Expertise is not something that once gained remains with the practitioner for always. With such rapidly changing knowledge and skill, only those in practice can actually retain their expertise. Hence, the teacher practitioners and mentors will retain credibility with learners for as long as they demonstrate their own expertise and professional knowledge in working with their mentees and students.

Conclusion

This chapter has opened up the debate about postmodernity, although it has not attempted to enter into the arguments. It recognizes the direction in which higher education is moving in countries that modernized with the Enlightenment. It demonstrates quite clearly that teacher practitioners and mentors, successors to the apprentice masters, are reflections of the age in which we live. They are a significant feature in professional preparation and continuing education – they are the experts sharing their knowledge, skills and attitudes with others.

Suggested further reading

The following books are suggested for readers who wish to pursue some of the topics mentioned in this book. Naturally, any list is bound to be selective, but it has been restricted to 24 books so that the reader will feel able to make a reasonable selection.

Alsop, A. and Ryan, S. (1996) *Making the Most of Fieldwork Education: A Practical Approach*. Cheltenham: Stanley Thornes (Publishers) Ltd.
> This book is intended to help student therapists maximize their learning in fieldwork placements. It is also useful to educators who work in these placements and who act as mentors and supervisors of students.

Boud, D. (ed.) (1985) *Problem Based Learning in Education for the Professions*. Sydney: Higher Education Research and Development Society of Australia.
> This book is relevant for all forms of professional education and it examines the theory and practice of problem-based learning.

Burnard, P. (1989) *Teaching Interpersonal Skills: A Handbook of Experiential learning for Health Professionals*. Cheltenham: Stanley Thornes (Publishers) Ltd.
> This book provides a guide to using experiential learning methods to teach interpersonal skills, supplying a theoretical explanation and details of how to organize and run experiential learning groups.

Butler, B. and Elliott, D. (1985) *Teaching and Learning for Practice*. Aldershot: Gower.
> This book has been produced in conjunction with *Community Care*. It is a useful handbook for social work professionals and educators who work in the practice situation.

Butterworth, T. and Faugier, J. (eds) (1992) *Clinical Supervision and Mentoring in Nursing*. Cheltenham: Stanley Thornes (Publishers) Ltd.
> A book of 17 chapters covering a variety of topics relevant to this subject It seeks breadth and introduces readers to a variety of practice situations.

Caldwell, B. and Carter, J. (1993) *The Return of the Mentor*. London: Falmer Press.
> This book, comprising 12 chapters, examines a variety of workplace learning experiences. Although it is not specifically aimed at health care professionals, it does provide a broad and interesting perspective, and guidelines for good practice.

Daloz, L. (1986) *Effective Teaching and Mentoring*. San Francisco: Jossey Bass.
This is a well-written book about mentoring in adult education. It provides a model for all educators.

de Tornay, R. (1987) *Strategies for Teaching Nursing*. Chichester: John Wiley & Sons.
This book is aimed at experienced nurse educators to help them formulate and meet educational objectives in their own teaching.

Glover, G. and Mardle, G. (eds) (1995) *The Management of Mentoring*. London: Kogan Page.
This book discusses policies about mentoring within a broader context. It contains case studies and looks at mentoring from a wider context.

Hinchcliffe, S. (1992) *The Practitioner as Teacher*. London: Baillière Tindall/Scutari Press.
A book providing a user-friendly guide based on an interactive personal style of presentation. It contains activities and places emphasis on reflective practice and experiential learning.

Hull, C. and Redform, C. (1996) *Profiles and Portfolios for Nurses and Midwives*. London: Macmillan.
A guide for the preparation of portfolios to meet UKCC requirements. It provides sufficient information to help teacher practitioners formulate their own profiles and for them to assist others do likewise.

Krill, D. (1990) *Practice Wisdom*. London: Sage.
A book examining a number of different aspects of practice in social work which would also be very useful for teacher practitioners.

McIntyre, D., Hagger, H. and Wilkin, M. (eds) (1993) *Mentoring*. London: Kogan Page.
This book examines mentoring in initial education. It raises interesting and relevant questions, and points to some areas of good practice and future trends.

Megginson, A. and Clutterbuck, D. (eds) (1995) *Mentoring in Action*. London: Kogan Page.
This is a practical book for managers in general. It uses case studies to help managers think about their organization as a learning organization. It is broad, practical and interesting.

Morton-Cooper, A. and Palmer, A. (1993) *Mentoring and Preceptorship*. Oxford: Blackwell.
An introduction to mentoring and preceptorship in nursing, citing some of the recent research. A good practical introduction to the topic.

Murray, M. with Owen, M. (1991) *Beyond the Myths and Magic of Mentoring*. San Francisco: Jossey Bass.
This book is based upon industrial practices in the USA. It adopts a clear practical approach. It would be an interesting book for health care professionals to read.

Ogier, M. (1989) *Working and Learning*. London: Scutari Press.
This book is aimed at qualified nurses who are required to provide an environment in which student nurses can acquire and practise nursing skills,

and trained nurses can continue to increase their knowledge and skills. Drawing on previous research studies, it links learning and working.

Quinn, F. (1995) *The Principles and Practice of Nurse Education* (3rd edition). Cheltenham: Stanley Thornes (Publishers) Ltd.
This book covers a wide range of education within nursing and health care. It is a combination of principles and practice and can be applied to a variety of settings.

Rogers, A. (1986) *Teaching Adults*. Milton Keynes: Open University Press.
A comprehensive coverage of major issues in teaching adults. It is aimed at lecturers as well as those who teach practice. It emphasizes the practice of teaching.

Rogers, J. (1989) *Adults Learning* (3rd edition). Milton Keynes: Open University Press.
This book has been well-used by educators of adults. It is clearly written and very practical.

Rowland, S. (1993) *The Enquiring Tutor*. London: Falmer Press.
This book examines the relationship between tutoring and professional workers on post-experience courses. It is a worthwhile book for all tutors who are concerned with the way that they relate to professional practitioners.

Schon, D. (1983) *The Reflective Practitioner*. New York: Basic Books.
This book has recently been published in paperback by Arena in Aldershot. Schon, has written a follow-up, *Educating the Reflective Practitioner* (1987), San Francisco: Jossey Bass. The book has become extremely popular and it should be read by all who embark upon teaching reflective practice.

Spouse, J. (1990) *An Ethos of Learning*. London: Scutari Press.
Based on an M.Sc. dissertation at the University of Surrey, this book demonstrates the conflict of competing priorities in the delivery of care and the acquisition of knowledge.

Bibliography

Alexander, M. (1983) *Integrating Theory and Practice.* Edinburgh: Churchill Livingstone.

Argyris, C. (1982) *Reasoning, Learning and Action.* San Francisco: Jossey Bass.

Armstrong, P.F. (1982) The 'needs meeting' ideology in liberal adult education, in *International Journal of Lifelong Education,* **1** (4).

Barlow, S. (1991) Impossible dream: Why doesn't mentorship work in UK nurse education? *Nursing Times,* **87.**

Barrow, R. and White, P. (eds) (1993) *Beyond Liberal Education.* London: Routledge.

Baskett, M. and Marsick, V. (1992) *Professionals' Ways of Knowing.* San Francisco: Jossey Bass.

Bateman, W. (1990) *Open to Question.* San Francisco: Jossey Bass.

Battle, S. and Salter, B. (1981) *Evaluation of the District Nurse Course (SRN/RGN),* 2nd Interim Report. Guildford: University of Surrey.

Baudrillard, J. (1988) The system of objects, in Prosser, M. (1988) op. cit.

Bauman, Z. (1992a) *Mortality, Immortality and Other Life Strategies.* Cambridge: Polity Press.

Bauman, Z. (1992b) *Intimations of Postmodernity.* London: Routledge.

Beard, R. (1976) *Teaching and Learning in Higher Education* (3rd edition). Harmondsworth: Penguin.

Belbin, E. and Belbin, R.M. (1972) *Problems in Adult Retraining.* London: Heinemann.

Benner, P. (1984) *From Novice to Expert.* Menlo Park, California: Addison Wesley.

Benner, P. and Wrubel, J. (1989) *The Primacy of Caring.* Menlo Park, California: Addison Wesley.

Berger, P.L. and Luckmann, T. (1967) *The Social Construction of Reality.* London: Allen Lane, The Penguin Press.

Bines, H. (1992) Issues in course design, in Bines, H. and Watson, D. (eds) (1992) op. cit.

Bines, H. and Watson, D. (1992) *Developing Professional Education.* Milton Keynes: Open University Press.

Blank, W. (1982) *Handbook for Developing Competency-Based Training Programs.* Englewood Cliffs, New Jersey: Prentice Hall.

Bligh, D.A. (1971) *What's the Use of Lectures?* Exeter: D.A. and B. Bligh, Briar House.

Bloom, B.S. (ed.) (1956) *Taxonomy of Educational Objectives, Book 1: Cognitive Domain.* London: Longman.

Boone, E. (1985) *Developing Programs in Adult Education*. Englewood Cliffs, New Jersey: Prentice Hall.

Botkin, J., Elmandjra, M. and Malitza, M. (1979) *No Limits to Learning: Bridging the Human Gap*. London: Pergamon.

Boud, D., Keogh, R. and Walker, D. (1985) *Reflection: Turning Experience into Learning*. London: Kogan Page.

Bowles, S. and Gintis, H. (1976) *Schooling in Capitalist America*. London: Routledge & Kegan Paul.

Bradshaw, J. (1972) The concept of social need, *New Society*, 30 March.

Bruner, J. (1977) *The Process of Education* (2nd edition). Cambridge, Mass.: Harvard University Press.

Buber, M. (1947) *Between Man and Man*. London: Kegan Paul, Trench, Truber & Co.

Buber, M. (1959) *I and Thou*. Edinburgh: T. & T. Clark.

Cardwell, B. and Carter, M. (eds) (1993) *The Return of the Mentor*. London: Falmer Press.

Carruthers, J. (1993) The principles and practice of mentoring, in Cardwell, B. and Carter, M. (eds) (1993) op. cit.

Carter, M. (1993) Coaching trainers for workplace performance, in Cardwell, B. and Carter, M. (eds) (1993) op. cit.

Chickering, A.W. and associates (1981) *The Modern American College*. San Francisco: Jossey Bass.

Coombes, P.II. and Ahmed, M. (1974) *Attacking Rural Poverty: How Non-Formal Education Can Help*. Baltimore: Johns Hopkins University Press.

Cooper, C.L. (ed.) (1976) *The Theories of Group Processes*. London: John Lilley & Sons.

Costin, F. (1972) Lecturing versus other methods of teaching: A review of research, *British Journal of Educational Technology*, **13** (1).

Cross, K.P. (1981) *Adults as Learners*. San Francisco: Jossey Bass.

Delors, J. (chairman) (1996) *Learning: The Treasure Within*. Paris: Unesco Publishing.

Daloz, L. (1986) *Effective Teaching and Mentoring*. San Francisco: Jossey Bass.

Davies, I.K. (1971) *The Management of Learning*. London: McGraw-Hill.

Davies, I.K. (1976) *Objectives in Curriculum Design*. London: McGraw-Hill Book Company.

Davis, B. (ed.) (1983) *Research into Nurse Education*. London: Croom Helm.

Davis, E. (1980) *Teachers as Curriculum Evaluators*. London: George Allen & Unwin.

de Tornyay, R. and Thompson, M.A. (1982) *Strategies for Teaching Nursing*. New York: John Wiley & Sons.

de Wit, P. (1993) *Approaches to Good Practice in Quality Assurance in University Continuing Education*. Working Paper No. 3, University Council for Adult and Continuing Education, University of Birmingham.

Dobby, J. (1981) *An Evaluation of the Procedures Used to Assess the Practical Work of District Nurse Trainees*. Uxbridge: Brunel University.

Dreyfus, H.L. and Dreyfus, S.E. (1981) The movement from novice to expert: What experience teaches, cited in de Tornyay, R. and Thompson, M.A. (1982) op. cit.

Eisner, E.W. (1969) Instructional and expressive objectives, in Popham *et al.* (1969) op. cit.

Eisner, E. (1985) *The Art of Educational Evaluation: A Personal View*. London: Falmer Press.

English National Board (1982) *Rules, Regulations, Notes for Guidance and Syllabuses for Courses*. London: ENB.

English National Board (1983) *Regulations and Guidelines for District Nurse Education and Training and Related Matters*. London: Panel of Assessors for District Nurse Training.

English National Board (1993) *Regulations and Guidelines Relating to Programmes of Education Leading to the Qualification of Specialist Practitioner*, 04/RLV. London: ENB.

Erikson, E.H. (1965) *Childhood and Society*. Harmondsworth: Penguin.

Eurich, N. (1985) *Corporate Classroom*. Princeton: Carnegie Foundation for the Advancement of Teaching.

Feigenbaum, E. and McCorduck, P. (1984) *The Fifth Generation*. New York: Signet.

Fish, D. and Purr, B. (1991) *An Evaluation of Practice-Based Learning in Continuing Professional Education in Nursing, Midwifery and Health Visiting*. London: ENB.

Fox, D. (1983) Personal theories of teaching, *Studies in Higher Education*, **8** (2).

Freire, P. (1972a) *Pedagogy of the Oppressed*. Harmondsworth: Penguin.

Freire, P. (1972b) *Cultural Action for Freedom*. Harmondsworth: Penguin.

Fretwell, J. (1979) *Socialisation of Nurses: Teaching and Learning in Hospital Wards*. University of Warwick: Unpublished Ph.D. thesis.

Fretwell, J. (1982) *Ward Teaching and Learning: Sister and the Learning Environment*. London: Royal College of Nursing.

Giddens, A. (1990) *The Consequences of Modernity*. Cambridge: Polity Press.

Giles, H., MacCutcheon, S. and Zechiel, A. (1942) *Exploring the Curriculum*, Harper.

Guba, E. and Lincoln, Y. (1981) *Effective Evaluation*. San Francisco: Jossey Bass.

Habermas, J. (1972) *Knowledge and Human Interests*. London: Heinemann.

Hagerty, B.A. (1986) Second look at mentors, *Nursing Outlook*, **34** (1), pp 16–24.

Hamilton, D. (1976) *Curriculum Selection*. London: Open Books.

Harrow, A.J. (1972) *A Taxonomy of the Psychomotor Domain*. New York: McKay.

Hartree, A. (1984) Malcolm Knowles' Theory of Andragogy: A critique, *International Journal of Lifelong Education*, **4** (2).

Harvey, D. (1989) *The Condition of Post-Modernity*. Oxford: Blackwell.

Heller, A. (1984) *Everyday Life*. London: Routledge & Kegan Paul.

Heller, A. (1988) *General Ethics*. Oxford: Blackwell.

Heron, J. (1981) *Assessment*. British Postgraduate Medical Federation, University of London and Human Potential Research Project, University of Surrey.

Hilgard, R.E. and Atkinson, R.C. (1967) *Introduction to Psychology* (4th edition). New York: Harcourt Brace Jovanovich.

Hirst, P.H. and Peters, R.S. (1970) *The Logic of Education*. London: Routledge & Kegan Paul.

Honey, P. and Mumford, A. (1986) *Manual of Learning Styles*. Berkshire: Honey and Mumford.

Houle, C.O. (1972) *The Design of Education*. San Francisco: Jossey Bass.

Howe, M.J.A. (ed.) (1977) *Adult Learning*. Chichester: John Wiley & Sons.

Illich, I. (1977) Disabling professions, in Illich *et al.* (1977) op. cit.

Illich, I., Zola, I.K., McKnight, J., Coplan, J. and Shanken, R. (1977) *Disabling Professions*. London: Marion Boyars.

Jarvis, P. (1978) District Nurse Examiners – How do they score?, *Nursing Times*, 9 March.

Jarvis, P. (1979) Assessment of teaching, *Journal of Community Nursing*, April.

Jarvis, P. (1983a) *Professional Education*. London: Croom Helm.

Jarvis, P. (1983b) *Adult and Continuing Education: Theory and Practice*. London: Croom Helm.

Jarvis, P. (1987) *Adult Learning in the Social Context*. London: Croom Helm.

Jarvis, P. (1992) *Paradoxes of Learning*. San Francisco: Jossey Bass.

Jarvis, P. (1994) Learning practical knowledge, *Journal of Further and Higher Education*, **18** (1).

Jarvis, P. (1995a) *Adult and Continuing Education: Theory and Practice* (2nd edition). London: Routledge.

Jarvis, P. (1995b) Teaching and learning: Transaction or moral interaction, *Studies in the Education of Adults*, **27** (1).

Jarvis, P. (1997) *Ethics and Education for Adults*. Leicester: NIACE.

Jarvis, P. and Gibson, S. (1980) *The Education and Training of District Nurses SRN/RGN: An Evaluation of the Implementation of the 1976 Curriculum in Surrey (October 1978 – August 1979) – An Interim Report*. Guildford: University of Surrey.

Jarvis, P. and Gibson, S. (1981) An investigation into the validity of specifying 5 O-levels in the General Certificate of Education as an entry requirement for the education and training of district nurses, *Journal of Advanced Nursing Studies* **6**.

Kadushin, A. (1976) *Supervision in Social Work*. New York: Columbia University Press.

Kelly, A.V. (1977) *The Curriculum Theory and Practice*. London: Harper & Row.

Kelly, A.V. (1989) *The Curriculum: Theory and Practice*. London: Paul Chapman.

Kelly, G. (1963) *A Theory of Personality: The Psychology of Personal Constructs*. New York: W.W. Norton.

Kerr, C., Dunlop, J., Harbison, F. and Myers, C. (1973) *Industralism and Industrial Man* (2nd edition). Harmondswoth: Penguin.

Kerr, J.F. (ed.) (1968) *Changing the Curriculum*. London: University of London Press.

Kidd, J.R. (1973) *How Adults Learn* (2nd edition). Chicago: Association Press.

Kitchen, S. (1993) Preceptorship in hospitals, in Cardwell, B. and Carter, M. (eds) (1993) op. cit.

Knowles, M. (1980) *The Modern Practice of Adult Education* (2nd edition). Chicago: Association Press.

Knowles, M. (1984) *Andragogy in Action*. San Francisco: Jossey Bass.

Knowles, M. (1989) *The Making of an Adult Educator*. San Francisco: Jossey Bass.

Knox, A.B. (1977) *Adult Development and Learning*. San Francisco: Jossey Bass.

Kolb, D.A. and Fry, R. (1975) Towards an applied theory of experiential learning, in Cooper, C.L. (ed.) (1976) op. cit.

Kolb, D.A. (1984) *Experiential Learning*. Englewood Cliffs, New Jersey: Prentice Hall.

Krathwohl, D.R., Bloom, B.S. and Masia, B.B. (1964) *Taxonomy of Educational Objectives, Book 2 Affective Domain*. London: Longman.

Krech, D., Crutchfield, R.S. and Ballachey, E.L. (1962) *Individual in Society*. New York: McGraw-Hill.

Krill, D. (1990) *Practice Wisdom*. London: Sage.

Kumar, K. (1987) *Utopia and Anti-Utopia*. Oxford: Blackwell.

La Belle, T. (1982) Formal, nonformal and informal education: A holistic perspective on lifelong learning, *International Review of Education*, **28** (2).

Laschinger, H. and Boss, M. (1984) Learning styles of nursing students and career choice, *Journal of Advanced Nursing*, **9**, pp 375–80.

Laschinger, H. (1986) Learning styles of nursing students: Two clinical nursing settings, *Journal of Advanced Nursing*, **11**, pp 289–94.

Lave, J. and Wenger, E. (1991) *Situated Learning*. Cambridge: Cambridge University Press.

Lawson, K.H. (1975) *Philosophical Concepts and Values in Adult Education*. Nottingham: University of Nottingham, Department of Adult Education.

Legge, D. (1974) The use of the talk in adult classes, in Stephens, H. and Roderick, G. (1974) op. cit.

Levinas, E. (1991) *Totality and Infinity* (trans. A. Lingis). Dordrecht: Kluwer.

Levitas, R. (1990) *The Concept of Utopia*. London: Philip Allan.

Lewin, K. (1952) Group decision and social change, in Swanson *et al.* (eds) (1952) op. cit.

Lippitt, R. and White, R.K. (1958) An experimental study of leadership and group life, in Maccoby *et al.* (eds) (1958) op. cit.

Long, H.B. (1983) *Adult Learning*. New York: Cambridge Book Co.

Lyotard, J.-F. (1984) *The Postmodern Condition*. Manchester: University of Manchester Press.

Lyotard, J.-F. (1992) *The Postmodern Explained to Children*. London: Turnaround.

Maccoby, E.E., Newcomb, T.M. and Hartley, E.L. (eds) (1958) *Readings in Social Psychology* (3rd edition) New York: Holt.

McGregor, D. (1960) *The Human Side of Enterprise*. New York: McGraw-Hill.

McKenzie, A. (1990) *Learning from Experience in the Community: An Ethnographic Study of District Nurse Students*. University of Surrey: Unpublished Ph.D. thesis.

MacMurray, J. (1961) *Persons in Relation*. New Jersey: Humanities Press Ltd.

Mager, R.F. (1975) *Preparing Instructional Objectives*. Belmont, California: Fearon Publishers.

Mannings, R. (1986) *The Incidental Learning Research Project*. Bristol: Folk House.

Marcel, G. (1976) *Being and Having*. Gloucester, Mass: Peter Smith.

Marsick, V. (ed.) (1987) *Learning in the Workplace*. London: Croom Helm.

Maslow, A. (1968) *Towards a Psychology of Being* (2nd edition). New York: D. Van Nostrand Co.

Melia, K. (1983) Students' views of nursing: Doing nursing and being professional, *Nursing Times*, June.

Megginson, A. and Clutterbuck, D. (1995) *Mentoring in Action*. London: Kogan Page.

Merton, R.K. (1968) *Social Theory and Social Structure* (2nd edition). New York: The Free Press.

Mezirow, J. (1977) Perspective transformation, *Studies in Adult Education*, **9** (2).

Mezirow, J. (1981) A critical theory of adult learning and education, *Adult Education*, **32** (1), Washington.

Mezirow, J. (1991) *Transformative Dimensions of Adult Learning*. San Francisco: Jossey Bass.

Mills, H. (1977) *Teaching and Training: A Handbook for Instructors*. London: Macmillan.

Morton-Cooper, A. and Palmer, A. (1993) *Mentoring and Preceptorship*. Oxford: Blackwell.

Murray, M. with Owen, M. (1991) *Beyond the Myths and Magic of Mentoring*. San Francisco: Jossey Bass.

Nicholls, A. and Nicholls, H. (1978) *Developing a Curriculum: A Practical Guide*. London: George Allen & Unwin.

Nouwen, H. (1971) *Creative Ministry*. Garden City, New York: Doubleday.

Nyiri, J. (1988) Tradition and practical knowledge, in Nyiri, J. and Smith, B. (eds) (1988) op. cit.

Nyiri, J. and Smith, B. (eds) (1988) *Practical Knowledge*. London: Croom Helm.

Ogier, M. (1982) *An Ideal Sister: A Study of Leadership Style and Verbal Interaction of Ward Sisters with Nurse Learners*. London: RCN.

Ogier, M. (1983) The ward sister as a teacher resource person, in Davis, B. (ed.) (1983) op. cit.

Orton, E. (1981) *Ward Learning Climate*. London: RCN.

Paterson, R.W.K. (1979) *Values, Education and the Adult*. London: Routledge & Kegan Paul.

Polyani, M. (1967) *Personal Knowledge*. London: Routledge & Kegan Paul.

Popham, W.J., Eisner, E.W., Sullivan, H.J. and Tyler, L.L. (1969) *Instructional Objectives*. Chicago, Rand McNally.

Pring, R. (1993) Liberal education and vocational preparation, in Barrow, R. and White, P. (eds) (1993) op. cit.

Prosser, M. (1988) *Jean Baudrillard*. Cambridge: Polity Press.

Reich, R. (1991) *The Work of Nations*. London: Simon & Schuster.

Reilly, D. (1975) *Behavioural Objectives in Nursing: Evaluation of Learner Attainment*. New York: Appleton-Century-Crofts.

Reischmann, J. (1986) 'Learning en passant': the forgotten dimension. Paper presented to the American Association of Adult and Continuing Education. Hollywood: Florida.

Robinson, D. and Robinson, J. (1989) *Training for Impact*. San Francisco: Jossey Bass.

Robinson, J.J. and Taylor, D. (1983) Behavioural objectives in training for adult education, *International Journal of Lifelong Education*, **2** (4).

Rogers, C.R. (1969) *Freedom to Learn*. Columbus, Ohio: Charles E. Merrill Publishing Co.

Rogers, C.R. (1983) *Freedom to Learn in the Eighties* (2nd edition). Columbus, Ohio: Charles E. Merrill Publishing Co.

Rogers, C.R. and Freiberg, H.J. (1994) *Freedom to Learn* (3rd edition). New York: Macmillan.

Rogers, J. (ed.) (1977) *Adults Learning*. Milton Keynes: Open University Press.

Rogers, J. (1989) *Adults Learning* (3rd edition). Milton Keynes/Philadelphia: Open University Press.

Rowntree, D. (1977) *Assessing Students: How Shall We Know Them?* London: Harper & Row.

Ryle, G. (1949) *The Concept of Mind*. London: Hutchinson House, republished in 1963 by Peregrine.

Sargant, N. (1990) *Learning and Leisure*. Leicester: NIACE.

Schaie, K.W. and Parr, J. (1981) Intelligence, in Chickering, A.W. *et al.* (1981) op. cit.

Schon, D. (1983) *The Reflective Practitioner*. New York: Basic Books.

Schon, D. (1987) *Educating the Reflective Practitioner*. San Francisco: Jossey Bass.

Schutz, A. and Luckmann, T. (1974) *The Structures of the Lifeworld*. London: Heinemann.

Sheffler, I. (1965) *Conditions of Knowledge*. Chicago: University of Chicago Press.

Simpson, E.J. (1966) *The Classification of Educational Objectives: Psychomotor Domain*. Urbana, Illinois: University of Illinois.

Simpson, I.H. (1967) Patterns of socialization into professions: The case of student nurses, *Sociological Inquiry*, 37 (Winter).

Sloan, J. and Slevin, O. (1991) *Teaching and Supervision of Student Nurses During Practice Placement*. Belfast: The National Board.

Smith, M. (1977) Adult learning and industrial training, in Howe, M. (ed.) (1977) op. cit.

Smith, R. (1982) *Learning How to Learn*. Milton Keynes: Open University Press.

Srinivasan, L. (1977) *Perspectives on Nonformal Adult Learning*. New York: World Education.

Stenhouse, L. (1975) *An Introduction to Curriculum Research and Design*. London: Heinemann.

Stephens, M.D. and Roderick, G.W. (1974) *Teaching Techniques in Adult Education*. Newton Abbot: David & Charles.

Swanson, G.E., Newcomb, T.M. and Hartley, E.L. (eds) (1952) *Readings in Social Psychology*. New York: New York.

Taba, H. (1962) *Curriculum Development Theory and Practice*. New York: Harcourt Brace & World.

Tennant, M. (1986) *Psychology and Adult Learning*. London: Routledge.

Thorndike, E.L. (1898) Animal intelligence: An experimental study of the associative processes in animals, *Pychological Review Monograph*, **2** (8).

Thorndike, E.L. (1911) *Animal Intelligence*. New York: Macmillan.

Thorndike, E.L. (1913) *Educational Psychology: The Psychology of Learning* (Vol. 2). New York: Teachers College.

Thorndike, E.L., Bregman, E., Tilton, J. and Woodyard, E. (1928) *Adult Learning*. New York: Macmillan.

Trenaman, J. (1951) The length of a talk: Report of an enquiry into the optimum length of an informative broadcast talk for the adult student type of listener, cited from Legge, D. (1974) op. cit.

United Kingdom Central Council (1993) *Registrar's Letter 1/1993*. London: UKCC.

Van Hoozer, H.L. (1987) *The Teaching Process: Theory and Practice in Nursing*. Norwallk, Connecticut: Appleton Century Crofts.

Van Ments, M. (1989) *The Effective Use of Role Play*. London: Kogan Page.

Walker, A. and Stott, K. (1993) Preparing for leadership in schools: The mentoring contribution, in Cardwell, B. and Carter, M. (1993) op. cit.

Wheeler, D.K. (1967) *Curriculum Process*. London: University of London Press.

Yakowicz, W. (1987) Coaching: Collegial learning in schools, in Marsick, V. (ed.) (1987) op. cit.

Young, M.F.D. (ed.) (1971) *Knowledge and Control*. London: Collier-Macmillan Publishers.

Author index

Subject index